90 Days to Beautiful *Curly* Hair: 50 Dermatologist-Approved Tips to Un"lock" The Natural (or Relaxed) Hair of Your Dreams

90 Days to Beautiful *Curly* Hair: 50 Dermatologist-Approved Tips to Un"lock" The Natural (or Relaxed) Hair of Your Dreams

Crystal Aguh, MD

ISBN:978-0-578-35302-9

Dedication

*This book is dedicated to my daughter, Chizara.
May you always love and cherish your hair and
everything else about you.*

Table of Contents

Introduction

Why I Wrote a Book Just for Curly Hair

In my first book, I really wanted to make it clear that even though we think of different hair types from various ethnic groups as worlds apart, the principles of hair care are largely the same across curl patterns, the one big difference being that curly hair requires more TLC, so while treating straight hair nicely is great, for curly hair, it's a necessity. That being said, there are clearly very unique properties of curly hair that need to be specifically addressed. In my clinic, I treat various forms of medical alopecia, many of which are not associated with hairstyling practices at all. However, because curly hair is more prone to breakage than straight hair, about 50 percent of my alopecia visits involve a discussion about hair care practices and how to make sure the hair is healthy while the medical condition is being treated.

I realize that this is not a topic of discussion many women have with their doctors. The truth is, hair care is often seen as a purely cosmetic concern and is not emphasized in health visits. As an alopecia specialist, however, I have learned that hair breakage can often make medical hair loss look much, much worse and can often lead to misdiagnoses. I have had patients who have been diagnosed with permanent, scarring hair loss and have received painful injections in their scalp for years, only to be evaluated in my clinic where they learn that their hair *can* grow and their hair loss was a result of very severe hair breakage, a condition called

Acquired Trichorrhexis Nodosa. So, in some ways, hair care practices are of medical concern, as understanding the hair can save women the emotional and financial distress of a misdiagnosis.

For the purposes of this book, when I mention "curly hair," I am referring to hair that is naturally curly, whether it is worn in its natural state or relaxed. This is because, no matter how the hair is styled, hair that is naturally curly is much more fragile than hair that is naturally straight.

In my first book, I explained why curly hair is so fragile, and it is important to reemphasize that point here as well. One of the main reasons that curly hair requires more TLC is because it is less likely to be coated with sebum, the natural moisturizer produced by the scalp. Couple this with the fact that the hair growth rate of many women of African descent is slightly slower than other ethnic groups, the end result is that it is harder for many curly haired women to grow their hair past shoulder length.

The good news is that with the right instructions and a healthy hair regimen, it is possible to unlock your hair's maximum potential and reach lengths you may never have deemed possible.

The rules of my first book still apply today. Here is what this book will not do:

- It will not give you a super-secret tip to making your hair grow *faster*, even if you are able to get it to grow *longer.* How fast your hair grows is predetermined genetically and cannot be altered. If I ever do discover how to alter your predetermined genetic growth rate, I will certainly write a book for all of my loyal readers and retire somewhere on an island far away very, very rich.
- It will not change the natural characteristics of your hair. For example, if your hair is naturally low density, your hair will not suddenly become high density BUT this hair care regimen will make your hair fuller over time due to less breakage. Depending on who you are, this change may still be drastic, especially if you have a lot of room for improvement.

The good news is, in this book you will find fifty tips that will improve the overall health of your hair and help you grow your hair longer and stronger. Here's what this book will do:

- Give you healthy alternatives for your favorite styling practices.
- Give you a list of ingredients to look for in your hair products to make shopping easier.
- Teach you how to improve the strength of your hair and prevent damage.
- Help you understand the principles of moisturizing your hair so that your hair is stronger, shinier, and overall healthier.

Remember, all curly hair is considered fragile to some extent, and certain styling practices can make that fragility even worse. Three major factors that determine the likelihood of breakage and therefore the likelihood of growing the hair past the shoulders are:

- Curl pattern
- Hair thickness and density (fine/thin vs coarse/thick)
- Age

Together, these factors determine what I like to call, *hair resiliency.* Hair resiliency is a term I use to refer to the type of damage your hair can withstand before it breaks. As a general rule of thumb, thick/coarse hair in younger women tends to be more resilient than thin/fine hair in older women.

The first thing you should try and understand is your curl pattern, since I will be referring to it several times throughout the book. Realize, identifying your curl pattern is NOT an exact science. The most popular curl typing system divides curl types from 1A→4C with type 1 representing straight hair, type 2 representing wavy hair, type 3 representing curly hair, and type 4 representing coily or kinky hair.

The tips in this book are best suited for those whose curl types range anywhere from a 3A to a 4C.

You will see many different depictions of what it means to be 3A or 4C and everything in between. However, based on the numerous scalps I have examined, this is how I break down curl patterns (figure 1):

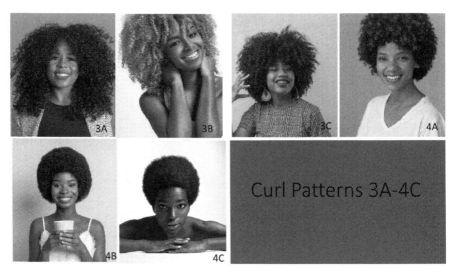

Figure 1: Curl patterns, from top left: 3A–4C. As the curl pattern tightens, the hair is naturally more fragile.

Additionally, many women have two different curl patterns on their scalp, which can complicate typing.

Looser curl patterns tend to be able to withstand more damage than tighter curl patterns. So that means in terms of decreasing resiliency 3A–3C>>>4A–4B>>4C, and 4C+ (see Chapter 1 for more on hair typing). If your hair is thin/fine, it is much less resilient than normal or high-density hair of the same curl pattern, meaning that fine/thin 4C+ natural hair is far and away most prone to breakage. In fact, paradoxically, women with this hair type may find they experience less breakage when the hair is texturized to a 4B or 4A-like curl pattern, as these patterns are less likely to become dry and are more easily moisturized and therefore less prone to breakage.

Lastly, as we age, hair naturally thins, and resiliency decreases over time. This means that styles you wore without issue when you were 22 may pull out your hair at age 42. Or similarly, if you grew your hair down your back when you were 12 and only washed your hair once a month, you may notice difficulty growing your hair past your shoulders with the same regimen twenty years later.

As you read this book, keep in mind where your hair falls on the hair resiliency curve. If you have more characteristics that make your hair prone to breakage, be prepared to make at least a handful of adjustments before seeing any improvement but also realize that the potential upside is greatest at this side of the curve.

Be patient. Be open-minded. Be prepared to uncover the hair of your dreams.

One

Embrace Your Curl Pattern

I am so happy to be talking directly to all my curly girls in this book. As you can tell, many chapters in this book are dedicated in some way to embracing your curl pattern. Curly hair is the most diverse hair type in the world. If your hair is straight . . . it's just straight. Some may have a slight wave to their hair, but for the most part, there are no additional special considerations when it comes to straight hair.

Curly hair is very different.

Recommendations for how to take care of 3A hair are totally different from 4A hair, which is still different from 4C hair.

And when it comes to curly hair, sometimes the grass seems greener on the other side. So before you dive any further into this book, I will say it again:

Embrace your curl pattern.

This is critically important if you are just learning how to take care of your hair. If you naturally have type 4C hair, it may be tempting to watch someone achieve a nice, moisturized twist-out on 4A hair. While your twist-out may still look beautiful, you may be discouraged when you find your hair does not behave in a similar way, and it may alter your expectations. It is really important to find examples of your exact curl pattern and density to set a realistic expectation.

Speaking of a 4C curl pattern, many women who think they are a 4C are truly more of a 4A or 4B and only call themselves a 4C because their hair feels difficult to moisturize or breaks easily. Moisture retention is honestly an issue with all type 4 hair, but often 4C seems like a catchall pattern, and it truly is not. In fact, there are many women who have hair much tighter than the average 4C depiction we see online, and I've grown to call this pattern 4C+.

A much more scientific study on curl patterns (see Appendix C) actually divided curl patterns into eight types. Curl type 8 is mostly found in Sub-Saharan (West and Central) Africa, whereas, in places like the United States/Canada, the tightest curl patterns tend to be more types 6 and 7. I see many women who are direct immigrants or first-generation immigrants from these regions who fall into this category. So, when I say 4C+, I am really referring to curl type 8. Unfortunately, there are very few media depictions of women with 4C+ hair, and for these women, it can be difficult to watch videos of women with so-called "4C hair" whose hair still seems easier to moisturize and define.

All of this is to say, half of the battle when it comes to taking care of curly hair is setting unreasonable expectations about hair care and styling options. Once you embrace your true pattern, it makes the journey much simpler and more enjoyable. Every head of hair is unique and has its own wonderful strengths, so spend less time on hair envy and more time loving your crown.

Two

Avoid Hair Care Tips from Those with Different Curl Patterns

I am such a believer in crowdsourcing for information. If you are new to your healthy hair journey, navigating this space can be hard. My hope is that this book will help in moving you along on your journey, but I also think places like Google, YouTube, and social media outlets like Instagram and TikTok (see Chapter 27) are great places to get tips too. One pitfall that must be avoided, however, is seeking advice from people with different curl patterns.

Having curly hair can be a constant "grass is greener" struggle. Women with looser curls wish they could create the elaborate braiding styles that seem to work best with 4C hair, and women with tighter curls wish they could achieve effortless wash and gos that women with type 3 hair achieve with ease.

Sometimes there are societal pressures at play as well. The reality is, society embraces looser curl patterns more readily than tighter curl patterns, and often, these are the curl patterns depicted when people refer to "beautiful" natural hair.

We are still working on a society that truly embraces all curl patterns, but don't let that be the reason you end up getting frustrated on your journey! Treating your hair like it's a 3C pattern when it's more like a 4B can lead to dryness and breakage. Additionally, realize that styles like well-defined twist-outs and braid-outs will look different on thin hair compared to hair that is fuller.

Remember, there is more diversity in hair types among women with curly hair than in women with straight hair. Take the time to source out and appreciate the styles that mirror your hair type. In the long run, you will be happy that you did!

(hair)

[Quiz Hour]

(~~non-coloring~~)

① What ~~a~~ Shampoo is best, for you 6 or you

& ~~for~~ your hair type?

① ~~②~~ What hairspray etc..

③ What ~~coloring shampoo,~~ etc.

② ~~③~~ ~~④~~ What hair conditioner is etc

③ ~~④~~ What combination of shampoo & conditioner is ~~best~~ best for your hair type

Three

Don't Underestimate the Effort to Go Natural

B elieve it or not, I have women who schedule appointments with me, a physician, to walk them through transitioning to natural hair. I politely tell them that I appreciate the compliment but that is absolutely not my lane! I am a physician, and in my clinic, I treat medical hair loss. Because hair care is often intertwined in the discussion of hair loss, I feel it is important to educate women on the science of hair care, as I am doing in this book. It is important for women to understand what their hair needs so we can be empowered to make decisions about our hair, whether it be at home or at a salon.

But I am not a stylist. Full stop. I cannot tell you which styles are going to frame your face better or if you would look better with a straw set or a flexi rod set. So much of styling comes down to personal preference.

In fact, I have my own stylist, and I don't know what I would do without her.

That being said, the sheer thought of transitioning to natural hair is so monumental that a part of me understands why some women would think it falls under the umbrella of a medical issue (again, it doesn't).

If you are a woman with type 4 hair in your thirties and forties and you have either a) been relaxed your entire life or b) hidden your hair in extensions for most of your life, then deciding to wear your hair natural is going to be a BIG transition. Please, please don't underestimate this.

Taking care of natural hair requires consistent hands-on effort from you. Many women with relaxed hair have a standing two-week appointment to get their hair washed by their stylist and may not require additional handling between appointments. Similarly, women who mostly wear extensions have a braider that they see every six weeks, who washes their hair immediately prior to installing their braids (later I will tell you why both of these approaches are not ideal).

This outsourcing of hair care is simply not feasible with natural hair. While yes, you can (and probably should) have a natural hairstylist that you see every few weeks/months, you will still need to get comfortable moisturizing your own hair in between visits if you want to maximize its health.

It is important to have a list of products ready to go as well as a well-thought-out plan about the transition to natural. Here is a list of staples that everyone going natural should own to start with:

- Shampoo
- Deep conditioner
- Rinse out Conditioner
- Leave-in Conditioner
- Moisturizing oil
- Styling cream

These products don't have to be expensive and can be purchased in large quantities that will last you several months. The bottom line is you want to be prepared *before* you transition to natural hair.

If you have spent most of your life in extensions, you will likely have damage that needs to be cut away first. If you have been relaxed, think about whether you want to "big chop," or if you want to slowly cut away relaxed ends.

But whatever you do, don't jump into being natural without having a plan first. This will save you significant frustration down the road.

Four

For Type 4 Hair: What it Takes to Grow Long, Natural Hair

O ne of the most common complaints I hear in my office is "my hair won't grow." When I hear the dreaded "my hair doesn't grow," it usually comes from women who notice that they have a particularly stubborn patch of hair on their scalp that always remains short. Oftentimes, this is the part of the scalp closest to the neck, but occasionally it's all over. If the breakage is just limited to one area, it is usually the portion of the scalp with the tightest curl pattern and the one that is hardest to moisturize. I am dedicating this chapter specifically to women with type 4 hair because this extent of breakage is much less common in type 3 hair.

The first thing I remind women who mention that their hair does not grow is this: "If you were to put in box braids today, six weeks from now would it look like you got it done yesterday, or would you have new growth?"

At this point, the light bulb usually goes off. *Of course* you would have new growth. Because the issue with curly hair is not whether the hair grows, it is actually *keeping* the hair that you have. For the most part, if you are living and breathing, the skin cells on your scalp are turning over, and as a result, you are producing new hair (the exception being a few forms of scarring hair loss, which are fortunately not too common).

But think about this. Imagine you are living in Sub-Saharan Africa 10,000 years ago with 4C+ hair. You are in a hot climate with no hair products or hair tools. What would you want your hair to do? Well, you would want it to grow upwards and not down because having hair resting on your shoulders would make you feel hot. In fact, you would love for it to naturally break off before hitting your shoulders to ensure this is the case. You would want it to be relatively low density, to make it easier for the scalp to cool. Finally, you would never want it to lay flat on your head, even if it is wet, because this would trap heat. Isn't 4C hair magical in this way?

Now consider those who lived 10,000 years ago in Northern Europe with the same issue—no hair products or styling tools. Well, in this case, you would want hair that would grow to long lengths, even if it is never taken care of, because this long hair provides extra heat for the body. You would want the hair to be denser to help trap heat in cold weather. Generally, it would also be preferable for the hair to lay flat on the head to help with this heat trapping.

Well, fast forward 10,000 years later, and long hair is associated with femininity and now women all over the world want long hair. Many women with type 4 hair assume that by going natural, their hair will suddenly be long and thick with minimal effort, but this is simply not what this hair type is designed to do.

Type 4 hair is glorious, and it is perfect, based on the evolutionary advantage it is designed to give, but it is not designed to grow long—without a TON of help.

Think about the amount of effort required to overcome something that is supposed to give you an evolutionary advantage. It requires a lot of time and effort. Fortunately, many of the techniques to achieve longer hair will be discussed later in this book. If you have type 4 hair and have made the decision to go natural, keeping your hair as moisturized as possible, with regular trims (!!), is critical to achieving your hair goals. If your hair is type 4C or beyond, this is a non-negotiable to healthy hair, as even one bad week could lead to enough breakage to set you back months in hair growth.

So, here are some tips if you are noticing no change in hair length over months to years:

1. Make sure you are deep conditioning every week. This is key to making sure your hair is moisturized for extended periods of time (see Chapter 11).
2. Use a leave-in conditioner regularly. If you are prone to dry, brittle hair, this likely means three to five times per week (see Chapter 20).
3. Devise your hair care regimen based on your tightest curl pattern. If your hair is mostly 4B, but the broken patch is more like a 4C, then you need to change your entire regimen to cater to that one area. The remainder of your hair will still thrive from this more aggressive hair care routine.
4. Trim your hair! I cannot stress this enough. I realize it seems counterintuitive to cut your hair when your goal is for longer hair, but if it's not gaining length, split ends are likely a contributing factor (see Chapter 29).
5. Avoid frequent use of extensions, including wigs. Wigs can dry out your hair, reversing all of the gains from your deep conditioner (see Chapter 33). In turn, this leads to more breakage. Similarly, extensions prevent you from performing frequent intensive conditioning treatments, which also are critical. There are certainly *some* exceptions. Sometimes, if women are complaining of breakage and never wear extensions or wigs but are constantly grooming their hair, then a short stint in large box braids with frequent care can actually be helpful. It is important to know if you have a hair type that will be suitable for extensions before employing this strategy (see Chapter 31).

Keep reading to learn how to devise your own hair care routine with enough helpful tips to help your hair grow as long as possible.

Five

Choose the Healthy Hair Path That is Right for You (Natural Versus Relaxed Hair)

If you read my first book, then you know that I generally do not have a preference when it comes to natural versus relaxed hair. Both hair types can be very damaged and both hair types can be completely healthy. Additionally, while there are a lot of myths surrounding chemical relaxers, there are no medical conditions definitively tied to relaxer use, aside from the potential for scalp burns, which is a very real risk if not applied correctly. The ingredients found in relaxers are actually quite similar to the ingredients found in hair dyes, which, again, are not tied to any medical conditions, but people seem to feel more comfortable using them for whatever reason.

So, let's go through some of the pros and cons of being natural or relaxed.

NATURAL HAIR
Pros

- Avoids the use of chemicals associated with a relaxer
- Hair maintains inherent strength because it is not weakened by a relaxer

- When healthy, hair tends to be fuller, which is especially important if the hair is naturally fine

Cons

- Harder to moisturize, which can lead to more breakage (this is less of an issue with type 3 hair, more of an issue with type 4 hair)
- Requires more time and effort to keep healthy (regular wash sessions are a must!)
- Requires more time and attention between stylist appointments to maintain (truly a hands-on approach)

RELAXED HAIR
Pros

- Requires less styling time
- Retains moisture more easily between washing sessions (this can mean less breakage if your hair issues are primarily related to dryness, as in 4C and 4C+ types)
- Shorter wash sessions

Cons

- Process of relaxing weakens the hair, requiring consistent use of protein treatments
- No-lye products buildup on the hair causing severe breakage
- Potential for scalp burns or hair loss if applied incorrectly
- Hair can appear overly thin on women with low-density hair

Ultimately, my approach to hair care recommendations is identical for natural and relaxed hair because I strive to encourage optimal hair care approaches. I still recommend washing once weekly, regular use of light protein treatments to boost strength, leave-in conditioners during the week, and regular trims. Having relaxed hair does not mean you get to skip out on hair care, but certainly, the hair responds differently to the same regimen.

I have met many women who go natural because they feel that it is "the right thing to do," only to then commit themselves to a lifetime of wigs and braids because they are not prepared to take care of natural hair, or they do not get the results they are looking for. I have met other women who choose to go natural but cannot let go of the idea of straight hair, and so they begin to flat iron their hair multiple times per week and get more breakage than ever before. It is important to pick a hair path based on what makes sense for you. Ultimately, hair thrives most when it is worn out and not tied up in extensions or overly heat-styled.

If you are looking for full hair, have a few issues moisturizing it, and love curly styles, then going natural is likely better for you. If you are busy and do not have the time to devote to hair care during the week and prefer to wear your hair straight, then relaxed hair is likely a better option. Choose your path without the impact of outside influence, then your healthy hair journey can truly begin.

Six

Save Your Money: No More Miracle Potions, Serums, or Vitamins

If you are reading this book, it is likely because you have experienced hair breakage or damage along the way. In curly hair types, breakage (often from dry, damaged hair) can be so severe that it exposes the scalp. This is not a *true* alopecia in the medical sense, it's just a result of sub-optimal hair care. And if you're curly, whether you're wearing it natural or relaxed, hair care must be optimal at all times.

However, if your social media is anything like mine, then you are inundated with numerous hair vitamins, serums, and potions proclaiming an ability to "grow hair" and "reverse alopecia." Well, wouldn't that be nice? I would love it if I could just take a couple of vitamins and have thick, long, luscious hair. Haven't we all hoped for this at least once?

Unfortunately, this is not a realistic expectation.

Why not?

Well, for starters, very few vitamins or oils have ever been associated with hair growth, and the ones that have are for very specific conditions (see Chapters 43, 44, and 49). But hair loss can be so emotionally draining that companies prey on consumers and convince them that if they spend tens or hundreds of dollars, all of their hair issues will go away.

Don't let that be you.

What we will be working on in this book are tactics to strengthen your hair to enhance length retention. Hair is always growing, it's just more difficult to sustain length because of the fragility and unique needs, but we are going to address all of that. So, save your money and continue reading about ways to transform your hair . . .

Seven

Break Out of the "Ethnic" Hair Aisle

I am sure this topic, which I also touched on in my first book, is still one of my most controversial. As I mentioned in the introduction, there is such a focus on race and ethnic group that when it comes to hair care, many feel like it is impossible that a product designed for blonde hair could be a staple product for a Black woman with curly hair. However, the best indicator as to whether a product will work for you is the ingredients list, not the model on the bottle or the aisle you find it in.

It is time to think outside of the box.

Hair companies realize that marketing their products to certain demographics can make consumers feel "special," when in reality, it's just a ploy.

When searching for hair products, you should feel comfortable ignoring these marketing ploys and pay attention to the ingredients that are safe for your hair. Generally speaking, products marketed toward "ethnic" hair and those marketed as "color-safe" tend to have gentler, fewer damaging ingredients than those marketed for normal hair, so these can often be interchangeable. This is because hair that is curly and has been colored are both more prone to damage. You will see in my product recommendations list products that are marketed toward women of all ethnic groups (see Appendix B).

By the time you are finished, you should feel comfortable walking down any beauty aisle and choosing the products that make the most sense for you.

Eight

Hair Cleansing: What Curly Girls Need to Know

I believe that a healthy hair care regimen begins with a proper cleansing regimen, especially for women with damaged hair. I want to start with the very basics. As I have mentioned earlier, curly hair is inherently more fragile, at every twist of the curl. Additionally, it becomes dry more easily than straight hair. Think about a twig on a branch; it is much easier to snap if it is dry and brown in the center than if it is thick and green. A big reason why curly hair is drier than straight hair is the lack of sebum coating.

Sebum is the natural moisturizer produced by the scalp. In people with straight hair, sebum finds its way down the entire length of the hair shaft daily from simply stroking and brushing the hair. Not only is sebum a great moisturizer, but it is also a great protector of the hair shaft. Well, try and imagine how difficult it is for sebum to find its way down every twist and turn of a curly hair strand. The more twists, the less likely sebum is to coat the entire strand, leaving the tips of the hair most vulnerable to damage.

One of the reasons women with short curly hair don't experience the breakage that happens to long curly hair is because sebum can generally coat the first couple inches of hair with no problem. But as the hair grows, the likelihood that sebum coats the entire strand decreases, especially if you have more coils. The less sebum protection, the more breakage.

Couple this with the fact that the growth rate of many women of African descent is slightly slower compared to women in other racial groups, and the result is that it is harder for many Black curly-haired women to grow their hair past shoulder length.

Because sebum is also a strong attractor of dirt, women with straight hair feel more inclined to wash their hair daily, but this is absolutely unnecessary for women with curly hair and is also damaging.

I typically recommend curly girls start their healthy hair routine by washing their hair at least once a week, especially if your curl pattern falls in the 4B/4C range.

This allows the hair to get enough moisturizing sessions without stripping the hair too much. However, there is some flexibility here (as with all things). For example, curly girls with type 3A/3B hair may notice that their hair becomes greasy faster, and in this case, wash sessions two to three times per week may be necessary. Women with type 3C/4A hair may notice that while their hair does not feel greasy, they are able to maintain a moisturized feel for up to two weeks, so frequent washing is less necessary.

SHAMPOOS

Shampooing is the process of removing sebum and dirt buildup. I know what you are thinking: if your hair has low sebum protection, to begin with, why would you want to constantly work at removing it? Well, the short answer is, you definitely do not want to remove it often, but there is absolutely a role for regular shampooing as part of a healthy hair routine for curly hair. The earliest shampoos used on the hair were basic soaps that people used on their skin. These were not meant to have any properties to beautify the hair and certainly did not make the hair appear glossier. Their most basic function was, and still is, to remove dirt from the hair. We no longer use basic soaps to wash our hair but more complex shampoos, some containing multiple types of cleansing ingredients as well as conditioning agents and glossers to please the consumer.

All shampoos are composed of at least one primary ingredient called a surfactant. A surfactant is designed to be attracted to both dirt and water, allowing dirt to be washed out easily while bathing. There are many different types of surfactants marketed today but they generally fall into one of four classes: anionic, cationic, non-ionic, and amphoteric. Don't worry, I know most of you have nightmares from your chemistry class, so I will keep this brief and limit it to what you need to know to keep your hair beautiful.

ANIONIC SURFACTANTS

The most common surfactant used is an anionic surfactant. This type of surfactant is superb at removing dirt from the hair, making it ideal for cleansing. Unfortunately, anything that is great at removing dirt is often great at removing protective sebum as well. For those with straight hair, this is not much of an issue because sebum is produced daily and can recoat the hair quickly, but for curly or damaged hair thirsting for moisture, it can lead to less than desirable results.

Anionic surfactants get their name from the fact that they are *negatively* charged. Our hair hates a negative charge, and when shampoo is applied to the hair, the negative charge is left behind. So, if you forget to use conditioner, you will notice hair that is dry, brittle, and frizzy. To restore the hair's neutral charge, a conditioner that is *positively* charged is required. This is the reason why the two must be used together and shampoo cannot be used alone.

Almost all ingredients listed on your shampoo that contain the word "-sulfate" are anionic surfactants. So, technically, a sulfate-free shampoo is one that is reported to be free of sulfates, which can be harmful to the hair. However, a shampoo could still contain an anionic surfactant and be marketed as "sulfate-free". See the table below for additional anionic surfactants:

Anionic Surfactants
The products are the best at removing product buildup but can be drying. Use sparingly (listed from most harsh to least harsh)
Sodium Lauryl Sulfate Sodium Laureth Sulfate Sodium Lauroyl Sarcosinate Ammonium Lauryl Sulfate Sodium Myreth Sulfate Sodium C14-16 Olefin Sulfonate Disodium Laureth Sulfosuccinate

The most commonly used anionic surfactant, sodium lauryl sulfate (SLS), is considered the prototypical member of this class and is also believed to have the best cleansing ability. Likewise, it is also considered to be the harshest of all shampoo surfactants. This can be problematic, not only for women with curly hair but also for those with hair that has been heat-damaged, has been colored, or chemically styled.

Anionic surfactants are absolutely the most skilled at removing sebum, but if your hair isn't coated with much sebum, do you really need a strong, anionic surfactant-containing shampoo? Well, that brings us to the next topic . . .

SULFATE-FREE SHAMPOOS

Often, when companies label their shampoos as "sulfate-free," they are referring to the absence of SLS. However, there are many other anionic surfactants that can be nearly as damaging as SLS, including sodium laureth sulfate (SLES) or ammonium laureth sulfate (ALS). Sometimes shampoos will label themselves as sulfate-free if they are missing just one of these ingredients and sometimes if they are just missing any one of these three. There really is no standard.

I have a much stricter definition when considering if a shampoo is sulfate-free and that is whether or not it contains an anionic surfactant. This is a less confusing way to split shampoo ingredients.

If you are using a harsh anionic surfactant-containing shampoo, you will likely notice an immediate turnaround in your hair health just by making this one change. There are some reasons to use anionic-containing shampoos (see Chapter 10), but if you are committed to avoiding sulfate-containing shampoos, specifically those free of anionic surfactants, then keep reading for several ingredient suggestions.

Nine

Go Sulfate-Free with These Moisturizing Shampoo Ingredients

So, you've figured out that your sulfate-containing shampoo is working against you. Now what? Fortunately, there are several truly sulfate-free shampoos out there, but you really have to know what to look for. Remember, "sulfate-free" is mostly a marketing term and many shampoos may say they are "sulfate-free" but still leave your hair feeling dry. Below are some of my favorite non-anionic shampoo ingredients. When looking for a shampoo, you will want to make sure that these ingredients are toward the top of the list, so you know they are doing the heavy lifting in your cleansing routine.

Decyl Glucoside: While sulfate-containing ingredients come with a negative charge that can leave your hair feeling frizzy, decyl glucoside is in a class of ingredients called non-ionic surfactants. These shampoo ingredients have no charge at all, meaning they are less likely to leave your hair feeling dry. They work well with other shampoo ingredients and for that reason are a common ingredient in many popular shampoos. Decyl glucoside is one of the most common ingredients that you will find in a sulfate-free shampoo on the market, and for good reason.

Cocamidopropyl Betaine: This is another common ingredient found in sulfate-free shampoos. Unlike decyl glucoside, it actually carries two charges, a positive and a negative one, which cancel each other out to leave a neutral charge on the hair. As a result, shampoos with this ingredient tend to do less damage to the hair.

There is one other ingredient that you should be aware of because it looks like it is a harsh ingredient, when in fact, it is a gentle cleansing agent: **behentrimonium methosulfate**. Even though it has the word "sulfate" at the end of its name, behentrimonium methosulfate is not an anionic surfactant and is totally safe to use.

Below is a list of other sulfate-free ingredients you may find in your shampoos.

These ingredients are less likely to strip your hair for protective oils, and in the long run, can help minimize breakage.

Happy shopping!

Gentle Cleansing Ingredients
Benzalkonium Chloride Cetrimonium Chloride Cocamidopropyl Betaine Decyl Glucoside Lauryl Glucoside Stearamidopropyl Dimethylamine Cocamide MEA Disodium Cocoamphodipropionate Behentrimonium Methosulfate

Ten

Try This Gentle Sulfate-Containing Shampoo

I know what you're thinking, we just spent all this time talking about sulfate-free shampoos, just to start talking about using a sulfate-containing shampoo?? Don't call me crazy just yet; there actually are a few great reasons to KEEP a sulfate-containing shampoo as your go-to option for wash day. In fact, if you go to a salon, your stylist is most likely using a shampoo with a sulfate as its main ingredient. What gives?

Well, here are a couple of reasons to keep a sulfate-containing shampoo around:

1. As I mentioned previously, shampoos leave a negative charge on the hair, which is what attracts positively-charged conditioners to the hair (remember that opposites attract!). So, if you have even the slightest of a negative charge on the hair, your conditioner will *work better*. You're actually giving your conditioner more negative charges to hang on to and do its job. This is why salons typically use sulfate-containing shampoos, and if you think about it, some of your best moisturizing sessions happen at the salon. I have personally transitioned to using gentle sulfates each time I shampoo for this reason. Keep reading to see my favorite gentle sulfate ingredient below*.

2. Second, remember that these shampoos (anionic surfactants) do the best job at cleansing the hair. Many companies are starting to label sulfate-containing shampoos as "clarifying" shampoos just to emphasize the level of cleanliness that is achieved after using them. For my patients who prefer to wash only with conditioner, I recommend the use of a clarifying shampoo at least once a month. These shampoos typically have mid-level anionic surfactants in terms of "harshness." They can be helpful after removing braided or weaved styles that have been in place for several weeks. Many of my patients find it difficult to wash their hair on a regular basis when they are wearing extensions, and when the extensions are removed, there are usually weeks of buildup underneath. After shampooing with a clarifying shampoo, you should always follow with a rich conditioner to counteract its drying effects.

So, what is my favorite gentle sulfate ingredient?

C14-16 Olefin Sulfonate

This ingredient is found in a lot of shampoos that say they are "sulfate-free," but it is actually a gentle anionic surfactant. However, it is "anionic," aka negatively charged enough, to prime your hair for a conditioning treatment. Check out my list of product recommendations in Appendix B to find shampoo products with this ingredient.

Eleven

Deep Condition with Every Wash!

I cannot stress this enough. If you have curly hair, a major cause of breakage and lack of growth retention is dry, brittle hair. For this reason, the hair needs to be heavily moisturized at all times. The tighter the curls, the less flexibility you have on this.

Enter deep conditioners.

These are more intensely moisturizing conditioners that are designed to stay on the hair for extended periods of time, usually at least twenty minutes with a heat source. Ideally, you want your hair to feel moisturized for at least five to seven days after a wash. To achieve this, deep conditioners are a must. They are often designed to be used with heat, which allows the scales along your hair cuticles to lift up so that the conditioner can penetrate the hair shaft more deeply. Regular use of a deep conditioner helps temporarily mend split ends and provides more resistance to breakage from daily grooming. You can mix your deep conditioners with oils to provide an even more intensive moisturizing experience.

I strongly recommend women with curly hair to deep condition their hair during every wash session with a few exceptions (see Appendix A for a sample wash regimen):

1. If you wash your hair more than once weekly (i.e., fine 3A–3B hair, swim regularly, etc.) then you should not deep condition with

every wash. This could make your hair feel lifeless and too soft. Instead, limit deep conditioning sessions to once every one to two weeks and proceed with a more typical shampoo + rinse out conditioner combo if you wash your hair more frequently

2. If you have fine hair and notice that your hair feels limp very easily (this can be an issue, especially in the summertime), opt for a brief five-minute conditioning session that is slightly less intensive than a deep conditioning session but more moisturizing than a regular rinse out session.

Twelve

Co-Wash in Moderation

E ver heard of co-washing the hair? Co-washing was truly all the rage in the late 2010s. The idea behind co-washing is simple: if shampoos are so damaging (as discussed in Chapter 8), why not just use a moisturizing conditioner to wash the hair all of the time so the hair never becomes dry? This is not a bad thought. In fact, many conditioners contain mild, non-anionic surfactants that do have some cleansing properties, such as those listed in Chapter 9.

The issue with frequent co-washing is that, over time, the moisturizing capabilities of your conditioner decrease, and your hair becomes LESS moisturized the more often you use them. In my first book, I discussed the issue of co-washing to introduce the idea for many women who were not familiar with the practice. Fast forward years later, and I find that it is more likely to see women *overutilize* this approach as opposed to incorporating it as needed. So instead, I want to discuss the downsides of co-washing too much.

Thinking again to general chemistry—opposites attract. A shampoo places a negative charge on the hair and a conditioner brings in a positive charge. In fact, the more negative charge there is on the hair, the more attracted to the hair the conditioner will be. That means that shampooing the hair before conditioning makes the conditioner more effective. If your hair only sees a positive charge, over time it will start to repel more positive charge being added to it. Now, normal wear and tear that the hair experiences also introduces negative charges to the hair, but certainly not as much as a shampoo would.

Again, this is why co-washing is usually a practice done at home and almost never in a salon. When clients go to a salon for treatment, shampoo is almost always used first. Many people can agree that deep conditioning treatments in salons tend to be even more moisturizing than treatments done at home. That alone will tell you that shampoos are an important part of the process.

So, what is my recommendation?

While occasional co-washing is just fine and may temporarily help your hair feel more moisturized, the best practice is still just to stick with the regular shampoo + conditioner routine. If you feel like your conditioner is not doing enough, then I recommend trying other conditioners to get a better result. The exception to this advice would be women who swim or work out often and feel compelled to wash their hair much more often than the once-weekly routine I recommend. If you find yourself washing your hair more than three times per week, then introducing a co-wash session to replace a shampoo session is a great alternative to using a shampoo that often on curly hair.

Thirteen

Add Regular Protein
Treatments to Your Regimen

Most people reading this book will benefit from incorporating protein treatments into their regimen, some more than others. Protein
treatments and protein-containing conditioners are marketed toward
people with damaged hair and often use the words "repairing" or "recon-
structing" on the product label. As I am sure you are aware, our hair is
made of protein, specifically keratin. Over time, harsh styling habits break
down keratin, leaving the hair susceptible to breakage. If you were able
to look at a strand of hair under a special microscope, you would be
able to visualize small holes dotted throughout the hair strands. These
are the hair susceptibility points. Each twist of your curl is also a point of
susceptibility.

So, what is a protein treatment? Protein treatments contain small, or
hydrolyzed, proteins that are small enough to enter the hair shaft and
temporarily fill in these holes. This results in hair that is stronger and can
also lead to the appearance of fuller hair. The great thing is, the more
damaged your hair is, the better it works! That's because there are more
holes to fill in, meaning the difference will be more noticeable.

Protein treatments should be applied with heat, which lifts up the
outer portion of the hair, allowing the small proteins to penetrate more
deeply into the hair.

How often you use protein treatments depends on your hair type and damage:

- **Type 3A–3C healthy hair without chemical treatments:** Use a light protein treatment at home once every one to three months. Consider a heavy, salon-based protein treatment one or two times per year.
- **Type 3A–3C hair that has been colored, chemically treated, or heat damaged:** Use a light protein treatment at home every two to four weeks. Consider a heavy, salon-based protein treatment quarterly.
- **Type 4A–4B healthy hair:** Use a light protein treatment at home every two weeks. Consider a heavy, salon-based protein treatment quarterly.
- **Type 4C healthy and types 4A–4C damaged hair:** Use a light protein treatment at home every week (with every wash). See Appendix A for suggestions on how to incorporate a protein treatment and deep conditioner in a single wash session. If damaged, consider in-salon protein treatments monthly for three months, then quarterly.
- **Relaxed/texturized hair:** Use a light protein treatment at home every week (with every wash). Consider a heavy protein treatment quarterly.

For some people, protein treatments can make their hair feel dry and straw-like. If this is the case, you will need to follow with a deep conditioner or a really rich moisturizing conditioner. The benefits of a protein treatment only last until the next shampoo, but with regular use, you will experience less breakage, which will allow your hair to grow thicker and longer. Who wouldn't love that?

Fourteen

Pre-Poo Before You Shampoo

If you have never heard the term "pre-poo," it may sound like gibberish, but it actually is derived from the term "pre-shampoo," referring to everything you do before you shampoo your hair. As I mentioned in Chapter 8, the mere act of washing hair is dangerous in and of itself because it strips the hair of its protective coating.

Additionally, when water hits your hair strands, it causes immediate swelling of your hair. The scientific name for this process is "hygral fatigue." If your hair is weakened for whatever reason, rapid swelling can lead to sudden breakage as well as tangling of your hair. One effective way to combat this process is to apply an oil or conditioner to your hair immediately BEFORE you shampoo.

This preps your hair by moisturizing it before it gets stripped clean, minimizing the chances that it will become severely dry. There are so many ways to prep the hair with a pre-poo. Some women use a blend of carrier oils and apply it to damp hair, others apply conditioner to damp hair. Actually, hot oil treatment is a type of pre-poo (see Chapter 16).

If I had to pick one oil to use as a pre-poo, it would be coconut oil, though it needs to be used in moderation (see Chapter 15). Coconut oil is the only oil that's been shown to prevent hygral fatigue, but many oils likely work just as well. Avoid thick, viscous oils like castor oil as they are not that easy to wash away cleanly. Consider oils like grapeseed, jojoba, and olive oil instead if you prefer to avoid coconut oil. Try it during your next wash and consider making it a permanent addition to your routine if you like what you see!

Fifteen

Limit Coconut Oil to Wash Days

This is a tip that comes both from personal experience and from patient experience. Coconut oil has so many benefits, some of which I mentioned in the last chapter, but there are some drawbacks too.

First, let's start by talking about some of the benefits of coconut oil.

Coconut oil should be a staple on the beauty shelf for anyone reading this book and has more scientific data supporting its use for the hair than probably any other oil. Coconut oil is most helpful when used as a part of your hair wash routine because it has a unique chemical structure that allows it to penetrate deeply into the hair shaft. As a result, coconut oil has the ability to minimize the swelling and breakage that occurs when washing the hair (hygral fatigue, see Chapter 14). Unfortunately, while many oils may help with moisture retention, most have a molecular size that is too large to penetrate the hair shaft in the same way that coconut oil does.

Coconut oil can also help with your post-wash routine. As I mentioned before, washing the hair can lead to breakage and weaken the hair shaft. But coconut oil has actually been shown to minimize post-wash hair protein loss and improve moisture retention, thus leading to stronger hair.

Because of all this goodness associated with coconut oil, some women (including myself, in the past) have a tendency to overuse it. But using coconut oil too much can actually break the hair.

Why?

Well, because coconut oil works very similarly to a protein treatment. You can imagine that if you applied a protein treatment to your hair every day, eventually it would start to feel dry and brittle and eventually lead to hair breakage.

Some people like to add coconut oil to oil mixtures, which dilutes its concentration, so it is less likely to cause dryness and breakage. So, if you love your coconut oil mix, don't feel like you have to abandon it. The main point I want to drive home is that you should not use coconut oil on its own multiple times a week as it may do more harm than good. Like many other things, it is best when used in moderation.

I recommend using coconut oil as below:

1. Apply softened coconut oil to dampened hair and cover with a shower cap or warm towel for ten to fifteen minutes.
2. Shampoo and condition the hair as normal.
3. Apply coconut oil immediately after washing. Alternatively, you can apply a water-based (for thin hair of any curl pattern or normal density 3A–3C hair) or cream-based (thick, 4A–4C hair) leave-in conditioner to the hair if your hair is dry before applying coconut oil.

One last note: There are many different types of coconut oil available: virgin, refined, processed, unprocessed, and a combination of these four. I generally recommend organic virgin coconut oil whether it has been processed or not. You can play around with different varieties and figure out what works best for you.

Sixteen

Try a Hot Oil Treatment

If you are familiar with my content, then you already know that I love old-school hair treatments. Here's another one to try: hot oil treatments! Hot oil treatments have somewhat fallen out of favor because of the popularity of deep conditioning treatments but there is still a role for them in a healthy hair care routine.

Hot oil treatments can be done as pre-wash treatments or in place of a deep conditioner to help moisturize the hair. Alternatively, you can alternate between a deep conditioning and a hot oil treatment on wash days, depending on your preference. Hot oil treatments can be particularly helpful for women struggling to maintain moisture between wash sessions. In this case, both a hot oil treatment and a deep conditioner can be performed during the same wash session.

To warm your oil, place the bottle or container of oil directly in a warm water bath, or let it warm up naturally after application by covering your hair with a shower cap and warm towel.

Here are some of my favorite oils to incorporate into a hot oil treatment:

- Olive oil
- Grapeseed oil
- Jojoba oil
- Castor oil
- Avocado oil
- Coconut oil

You can mix and match these oils or use them individually. There are plenty of choices for hot oils, but what you will notice is that these oils are mostly carrier oils, not essential oils. Essential oils (like tea tree, peppermint, rosemary, etc.) are meant to have medicinal properties and are not fatty moisturizing oils, so they are meant to be applied directly to the scalp only (see Chapter 43). While you certainly can add a few drops of essential oil to your hot oil mix if you like, carrier oils should really be doing most of the work here.

Ready to try a hot oil treatment with your next wash? To start:

1. Dampen your hair with warm water.
2. Apply the oil mixture of choice to your hair (pre-warming is optional).
3. Cover your hair with a shower cap.
4. Cover your shower cap with a warm towel or scarf.
5. Let sit for 30–45 minutes before washing out. Follow with your normal washing routine.

Seventeen

Start Air-Drying Your Hair . . .

Air-drying is one of those styling habits that pretty much everyone recognizes is better for their hair but is rarely done as it is much harder to achieve a sleek, straight look typically accomplished by heating tools. Unfortunately, drying the hair with a heat styling tool pulls water out quickly and can leave bubbles in the hair strand that puts the hair at risk for damage.

Healthy hair burns at 451.4°F (233°C) but damage occurs at much lower levels than this. Like flat ironing, blow-drying the hair can lead to damage that builds up over time. If you are looking for fuller hair, adding air-drying to your hair regimen can drastically improve the strength of your hair.

There are many ways to air-dry your hair so that the end result is similar to blow-drying. These differ based on your natural hair type. A great place to find various techniques are social media sites like YouTube, Instagram, and TikTok, all of which house a treasure trove of hair tips (see Chapter 27). For now, just know that there are at least two ways to incorporate air-drying into your routine without eliminating heat-styling cold turkey.

1. Blow-dry your hair on a low setting until about 80 percent dry, then style. This is a great option for well-defined twist-outs and

braid-outs that have greater definition on hair that is slightly damp but not wet.

2. Or do the opposite: air dry your hair until is 75–85% dry, then blow-dry the rest on a warm or cool setting. This is a better option if you prefer to wear your hair in a straight style or a sleek bun

Committing to air-drying 100 percent is likely one of the most difficult tips in this book, mostly because it's difficult to completely replicate a look achieved with blow-dryers and flat irons. But if you can commit to air-drying even a little bit, your hair will thank you with more shine and density in the long run.

Eighteen

. . . Or Use a Hooded Dryer

Alternatively, if you are not a fan of air-drying your hair, a hooded dryer is a great substitute option. While they are more expensive than hand dryers, hooded dryers disseminate heat evenly all over the hair without causing any one area of the hair to get too hot. They are also perfect for achieving low manipulation styles such as roller sets and flexi rod sets. These styles tend to be easier to achieve if you are relaxed or have curl patterns 3A–4B. However, even if you do not plan on incorporating these styles, the benefit of cutting the time spent washing and styling your hair by half may be well worth the investment.

Another similar option is a diffuser. Though it is not a hooded dryer, a diffuser similarly helps distribute heat over a wide area, and by doing so, minimizes curl disruption and breakage. Diffusers are typically sold as attachments to hair dryers or can be purchased as a single styling tool.

Diffusers and hooded dryers are two ways to repurpose heat into a less damaging option. This can be great for those who have curly hair without significant damage. I also recommend these tools as transition options for those who are looking to eliminate the use of flat irons or frequently blow-dry their hair straight. These options allow you to achieve similar styles with much less damage.

Nineteen

Try a Hair Steamer

With all this talk about how terrible heat is for your strands, you would assume that hair steamers would be a terrible idea, but that couldn't be farther from the truth. While dry heat in the form of flat irons and blow-dryers can dry out your hair and lead to breakage, moist heat is actually great for your hair. Moist heat encourages the scales on your hair's cuticles to lift up and welcome more moisture, which leads to more resilience and less breakage.

Steaming treatments are ideal for hair that is very dry or damaged. If you are chemically styling your hair in any way (relaxers, bleaching, or dye), then a regular steaming treatment may go a long way. There are a few steamers that can be purchased online, but steaming treatments are also commonly done in salons.

1. To incorporate steaming into your regimen, apply your deep conditioner as you normally would during your hair washing session.
2. Instead of letting your deep conditioner sit under a shower cap alone, sit under a steamer (with or without a shower cap) to allow the moist heat to moisturize your strands. You can also steam your hair without a deep conditioner and just allow the moist water to moisturize your hair.
3. Rinse your hair out and proceed with styling as usual.

It's important not to overuse a hair steamer as too much of anything is bad after a while. Some people may notice that if their hair is over-moisturized, it feels limp and lifeless and will not hold on to styles well. Figure out your ideal steaming frequency by playing around with your regimen. To start, I would recommend trying steaming treatments monthly, then increasing the frequency as needed. You would be surprised what regular steam treatments can do for the health of your hair!

Twenty

Use a Leave-In Conditioner Multiple Times a Week

By now, I have hopefully convinced you of the wonders of condition-ers. Remember, conditioner is just synthetic sebum, so applying a conditioner to your hair is like doing the job your scalp is supposed to do. Leave-in conditioners are designed to keep your hair moisturized in between washes. For most curly-haired girls, adding a leave-in condi-tioner to your regimen is an absolute must. In fact, curly hair is so prone to dryness that simply relying on wash day to keep your hair moisturized throughout the week is often not enough. This is true for women with types 3 and 4 hair but most important for women in the latter group.

Leave-in conditioners contain some of the same ingredients that are found in regular conditioners but are not meant to be washed out. These are generally lightweight ingredients, so they do not weigh your hair down. There are water-based leave-in sprays (for those who require only minimal midweek moisture) and cream-based leave-in conditioners as well. I am calling them cream-based here just to distinguish them from lighter, water-based products, but these conditioners also have water as the initial ingredient. Unlike water-based conditioners, cream-based con-ditioners typically come in jars and feel thicker. Sometimes, the two can be used together to layer moisture, compounding their effect.

If your hair is on the drier side and you would like to incorporate leave-in conditioners, then I recommend the approach below based on your hair type. You will notice that there are multiple ways to incorporate leave-in conditioners depending on your hair type, so you may try a couple of techniques before deciding:

- Type 3A–3C hair (low or normal density): Apply water-based leave-in conditioner spray or lotion immediately after shampooing and conditioning to wet hair and repeat one to three times per week. It can be incorporated as part of a wash-and-go style. If so, follow with styling gel or curling cream
- Type 3C–4C hair (low or normal density): Apply a water-based leave-in conditioner spray or lotion followed by a cream-based leave-in conditioner or hair butter three to five times a week. ***Note, if wearing a low manipulation style like flat twists or cornrows between washes, multiple applications of a leave-in conditioner are not necessary as moisture is retained while hair is braided.**
- Type 4A–4C hair (high or normal density hair): Apply cream-based conditioner or butter after shampooing and conditioning followed by oil. Repeat the process five to seven times a week. Considerations for braided, low manipulation styles are as above.
- Type 4A–4C hair (fine/low-density hair): Apply water-based leave-in conditioner spray or lotion after shampooing and conditioning followed by oil. Repeat the process five to seven times a week. Considerations for braided, low manipulation styles are as above.
- Relaxed hair: Apply a water-based leave-in conditioner spray or lotion followed by a carrier oil) two to five times per week

When applying leave-in conditioners, make sure to focus on the ends of your hair, as this is the part of your hair that is least likely to be coated with protective sebum. Your leave-in conditioner should leave your hair feeling softer, and you should immediately notice less breakage from styling. If this is not the result you are getting from your leave-in, keep trialing different products until you are satisfied.

Twenty-One

Incorporate Glycerin-Rich
Leave-In Conditioners

O ne of the hardest things about having naturally curly hair, whether it
is relaxed or natural, is getting it to stay moisturized. Even with our
best efforts, the moisture from a deep conditioner may only last one or
two days.

I have already discussed the importance of using a leave-in conditioner multiple times a week, especially if you are a tightly curled natural
girl. Now I want to highlight one of my favorite leave-in conditioner ingredients: glycerin. Glycerin is a humectant, meaning that it helps pull in
moisture from the environment to keep your hair moisturized over time.

Glycerin is a primary ingredient found in many Jheri curl products,
which was a popular hairstyle in the 80s, though it is still in many products available today. To achieve a Jheri curl, a low potency relaxer (i.e.,
a texturizer) would be applied to loosen, but not eliminate, the curl pattern (see Chapter 40). To maintain a well-defined curl, fans of this style
were encouraged to use "Jheri curl juice" or "curl activators" to leave
the hair at peak moisturized levels throughout the day. These curl activators are simply water-based leave-in sprays loaded with high levels of
glycerin.

Even though Jheri curls are not as popular a style as they once were,
Jheri curl juice is still available and works quite well on natural and relaxed

hair. It is often much more moisturizing than classic leave-in conditioners, and the heavy glycerin content is particularly effective for hair prone to dryness, like 4B–4C hair natural or relaxed hair. Keep reading for additional suggestions on incorporating glycerin conditioners into your regimen.

Twenty-Two

Try a Greenhouse Treatment for Ultra-Dry Hair

For my 4B/4C ladies, dry hair is the most difficult part of the natural hair journey to overcome. If you have hair that responds well to a deep conditioning treatment, feel free to skip this chapter . . . you have all you need! But, if you're like many other women, even extensive deep conditioning treatments can fail to leave the hair feeling soft and moisturized for more than a day. If you fit this description, keep reading for a super helpful treatment tip!

Enter the greenhouse treatment!

This moisture-packed treatment is commonly referred to as a greenhouse treatment because the high levels of moisture one experiences are reminiscent of a greenhouse that houses plants. Similarly, in this treatment, you are exposing your hair to prolonged periods of moist heat. For this treatment you will need:

- Water
- A water-based leave-in conditioner, preferably with glycerin
- A shower cap
- Scarf

To start:

1. Dampen hair throughout with water.
2. Apply your leave-in conditioner of choice to your hair making sure no areas are left dry.
3. Wear a shower cap.
4. Cover the entire head with a silk or satin scarf and leave it on overnight.

When you remove your scarf and shower cap in the morning, you should notice intensely hydrated curls. If you're natural, please note that this will cause your hair to revert to its natural curl pattern if you previously had it in a stretched state. If you have no issue with curl reversion, you will love this simple, low-cost, ultra-hydrating treatment.

After completing your greenhouse treatment, you can proceed with normal styling, such as twists or braiding the hair. I *do not* recommend performing this technique more than once a week. Since it is so hydrating to the hair, more frequent applications can make your hair feel limp from being *too* moisturized (yes, there is such a thing!). However, when incorporated occasionally into your regimen, you should notice increased length retention over time and less breakage.

Twenty-Three

To LOC or LCO? Learn How to Incorporate Carrier Oils into Your Routine

While LCO versus LOC is not quite the "great debate" that natural versus relaxed hair is, many women tend to feel partial to one technique over the other. If you have never heard of these acronyms, let me break them down for you:

- L = Liquid (water, leave-in conditioner spray, or lotion)
- O = Oil (typically a carrier oil)
- C = Cream (thick conditioning cream or hair butter like shea butter, etc.)

We broke down the "L" and "C" parts in Chapter 20, so we will discuss carrier oils here.

Patients often ask me for recommendations about oils for the hair. For the record, there are no oils that have been proven to grow hair faster. However, applying oils to moisturized wet hair (after washing or after a leave-in conditioner) can help seal in moisture and thus prevent breakage, leading to longer, stronger hair. Most essential oils, which are often marketed as "promoting hair growth," are actually meant to be applied to the scalp only, and when applied to the hair, can actually worsen dryness and breakage (see Chapter 43). Considering this, I recommend moisturizing, fatty oils that won't dry out the hair. My favorites are:

- Jojoba oil
- Olive oil
- Grapeseed oil
- Argan oil
- Castor oil (only for very thick, coarse hair)
- Avocado oil

By curl pattern my favorites would be:

- Types 3A–3C: argan oil, jojoba oil
- Types 4A–4C: argan, grapeseed, olive, and avocado oils
- Type 4C/4C+ normal or high-density hair: olive oil, avocado oil, castor oil*
- Relaxed type 4 hair: argan, jojoba, grapeseed, olive, avocado oils

*Many women also apply castor oil to the hairline, eyebrows, or other thinning areas, and this can be done regardless of hair type. When used to seal in moisture throughout the hair, castor oil should be limited to thicker hair due to its viscosity.

The "L" in both "LCO" and "LOC" refers to some type of water-based liquid. On wash day, because your hair is already wet at the conclusion of your wash, you can consider that water to be your "L" and you go directly to the "C" or "O." "C" can also refer to a water-based leave-in spray or lotion, as mentioned in Chapter 20. Between washes, the "L" typically refers to a water-based leave-in spray or plain water that is spritzed onto the hair.

As far as the order of application, "LCO" refers to applying a cream or butter to wet hair and finishing with an oil, while "LOC" concludes with the cream or butter. Deciding the order of application varies from person to person and may even vary for you from season to season. For example, in the winter you may find that finishing with a butter or cream is more effective than in the summertime. Try both methods, with different products, until you find the combination that allows you to maintain moisture for as many days as possible.

Twenty-Four

Don't Apply Oils to Dry Hair

One confusing thing about oils is that they are not moisturizers, in the purest sense. Oils are meant to *trap* moisture to increase softness and minimize dryness over time. This can be a confusing concept for many, and I frequently hear things like, "I put castor oil/coconut oil/tea tree oil on my hair every day to make sure it stays moisturized." This is a big red flag and the first clue as to why the hair is mega thirsty.

This is because the same way that oil traps moisture from getting on the hair, it can also *prevent* moisture from entering, especially if it is a thicker oil.

Think about body oils; these are meant to be used right when you get out of the shower. When you apply it to skin that is already wet, it leaves the skin feeling ultra-soft. If you were to apply the same oil to dry skin, especially dry, ashy skin, the same oil would feel sticky and just sit right on top of the skin. The same premise applies to oils for the hair. I cannot emphasize this enough:

Always apply oil to wet or damp hair, never to dry hair

This one simple tip can transform your hair, even if you continue to use all the same products. Check out Chapter 23 for tips on how to layer your oil with other products to enhance moisture.

Twenty-Five

Consider Adding Hair Grease
to Your Routine

If you are a '70s or '80s baby, then you know all about hair grease. Whether it was Blue Magic, Super Gro, or Ultra Sheen, hair grease was a staple in most Black households. With the movement to embrace more natural products for hair care— like essential oils—hair grease has fallen out of favor with many women. But is hair grease really evil?

Many Black women experienced enviable length retention with the use of hair grease in the past, and I believe there is a definite role for hair grease in hair care. Hair grease is best used on type 4 hair, as it is less likely to make the hair feel "greasy" on this hair type and it is also best incorporated on wash day. Consider it an inexpensive alternative to more pricey hair products that are potentially less effective. If you are interested in reincorporating hair grease into your regimen, keep the following in mind:

1. Hair grease should be applied to the hair, not the scalp!
Some people believe that if they have flaking on the scalp, it means it's dry and therefore requires more oiling or "greasing." This is not true. Significant flaking of the scalp can be a sign of a condition called seborrheic dermatitis, aka "dandruff" (see Chapter 47). In some cases, greasing the scalp could make this worse in the long run. Additionally, hair grease is inert, meaning it contains no ingredients that are meant to have

biological activity. Therefore, greasing the scalp will not promote hair growth or "stimulate" hair follicles.

2. Apply to wet hair only and braid or twist into style

Hair greases often contain ingredients like petrolatum and mineral oil, which are emollients. Emollients are very effective at trapping moisture onto surfaces like the skin and hair, but they do not increase moisture. As I mentioned above, when applied to dry hair, they can prevent moisture from getting in, leading to more dryness in the long term. Make sure the hair is wet or damp prior to application, and after the hair grease is applied, the hair should be twisted or braided, which allows the moisture to settle in and not evaporate quickly. Some women even use hair grease to help them achieve well-defined twist-out styles as hair grease can provide a light hold.

3. Consider using a shampoo with a gentle sulfate if used regularly

Hair grease is a potent attractor of dirt. If you plan to use it on a regular basis, then incorporate the use of a mild sulfate-containing or clarifying shampoo to make sure your hair is clean between washes. Mild sulfate-containing shampoos can prime your hair for more powerful deep conditioning so this switch may not be bad in the long run. Check out chapters 8–10 for ideas on ingredients to be on the lookout for.

With regular use, you should notice increased length retention with the incorporation of hair grease. Leave a comment below and let me know what you think.

Twenty-Six

Switch Up Your Routine to Avoid a Winter Setback

M any of us have experienced it: cherished length retention occurring during the summer months only to experience dullness and break-age during the winter months. Curly hair is very fragile and requires a lot of TLC to thrive. For many curly girls, this means an adjustment in your hair care routine once the weather gets colder. In the winter, there is less moisture in the air, leading the hair to become drier and more prone to breakage. Well, there are many simple adjustments to make to your hair care routine in the winter to help avoid breakage:

1. **Minimize the use of extensions if you suffer from dry hair.** If you have tightly curled hair (think 4B, 4C, or 4C+), you may want to hold off tucking your hair in braids or weaves all winter. While it is certainly tempting to minimize hair care during the holidays, without weekly deep conditioning you may notice much more breakage when the extensions are removed.

2. **Switch up your deep conditioner.** In the summer months, humidity can be a big issue, so lighter deep conditioners may be preferable as they are less likely to wear your hair down and allow you to enjoy twist-outs. In the winter months, you need a deep conditioner that really packs a punch. Thick deep conditioners that come in jars are

more likely to moisturize well compared to conditioners in tubes or pump bottles.

3. **Add a glycerin-based leave-in conditioner to your daily routine.** This is another big difference between the winter and summer months. Glycerin pulls in moisture from the environment to give you more conditioning power, which can be a nightmare for summer twist-outs in a humid environment. In the wintertime, however, glycerin can really help magnify the softness you experience after your deep conditioner (see Chapter 21). Use it three to five times a week if your hair tends to be very prone to dryness.

4. **Get a trim!** I get it, you want to grow your hair longer and hold on to as much length as you can. However, this is not the time of year to hold on to split ends. These split ends can travel up your hair shaft and break your hair off much faster (see Chapter 29).

5. **Focus on low manipulation styles.** Styles that minimize the need to comb or brush the hair are ideal during this time of year. Think cornrows (without extensions), buns, flat twists, etc. One nice thing about the wintertime is that twist-outs and braid-outs are more likely to stay well defined in the low humidity winter weather.

Twenty-Seven

Leverage Google or YouTube for Styling Tips

It's not often that you hear a doctor refer patients to Google for help. While googling medical conditions can send you into a downward spiral of inaccurate self-diagnoses, googling hairstyling tips can be quite helpful for those who are newbies when it comes to styling their own hair.

To achieve healthy hair, it is important to get to know your hair inside out. Most of us cannot afford to have a stylist that takes care of our hair on a weekly, much less daily, basis, so part of your new hair care journey will have to involve getting up close and intimate with your hair.

For many who read this book, this will seem intuitive. After all, who doesn't take care of their own hair on a regular basis? The truth is, many of my patients have spent most of their lives doing minimal hair care in between stylist appointments. This means that when issues arise (their stylist moves, they take a financial hit, or a global pandemic arises), these women are at a loss for what to do. That is what eventually leads them to my office.

During these appointments, I do what I have done in this book—I give them a long list of hair tips and products that they should abide by to improve the health of their hair. When I get the deer-in-headlights look to terms like "weekly deep-conditioning" and "bi-weekly protein-treatments," that is when I know that a little more guidance is needed.

The great thing about platforms like Google and YouTube is that you can find a video on almost anything. If the beauty aisle is too daunting and you need to get a sense of a deep conditioner to try, you can find someone with similar hair that can detail their experience with the conditioner. If you need to figure out how to style your hair for a special event, there's surely someone on YouTube who can walk you through that too.

Of course, everything you find online must be taken with a grain of salt. Many of the most prominent YouTubers are paid to endorse hair and makeup products, so this may prevent an honest description of hair products. Influencers, the name given to men and women who get paid to use their social media pages to sell products, can make tens to hundreds of thousands of dollars by making videos like these, so the incentive to be biased is real. Also, very few of these influencers are actually trained in the area that they are considered experts, which is part of their appeal. People feel more comfortable taking advice from someone who they relate to—it's the power of the "if I can do it, anyone can" idea.

When approached correctly, Google and YouTube can be powerful tools used for good. It is so very important for every woman to feel comfortable taking care of her own hair. For many women, there is almost no way to achieve healthy hair without taking this step. It is of particular importance to curly-haired women who will need to apply conditioner every day to prevent breakage. If nothing else, I want women to walk away from this book feeling empowered with understanding that they control their own (hair) destiny.

Twenty-Eight

Find a Stylist Who Prioritizes Hair Health Over Appearance

A stylist is like a best friend, a therapist, and a doctor all rolled up in one. For many people, they are not just a stylist, they are family. This is why what I am about to say will be hard to hear:

> Stop right now and think about whether
> you should get a new stylist. Seriously.

Stylists can be amazing; they offer hand-holding and can teach you how to take care of your hair properly. They also have access to products that frankly are not available to the general public, which can result in beautiful results that you just can't seem to achieve at home.

But if you are dealing with recurrent hair breakage and thinning, your stylist may be part of the problem. Not on purpose, of course, but you know what they say about good intentions. Most stylists want to make their clients look their best, but this may come at the cost of the health of their hair. Not sure if you should be on the hunt for a new stylist? Answer the questions below:

1. On balance, does your stylist discuss ways to camouflage your thinning hair (weaves, clip-ins, updos, braids) instead of discussing methods to improve it?

2. Does your stylist continue to perform harmful styling habits (flat iron multiple times, use bleaching agents, leave relaxer on for longer than necessary) even when you repeatedly ask them to stop?
3. Does your stylist ignore you when you say you are experiencing pain from a styling treatment (i.e., burning from relaxer treatment or during flat ironing, tight extensions, etc.)?
4. When you ask for tips on taking care of your hair at home (including tips on how to do routine hair care that is also available at the salon), does your stylist refuse to teach you and insist you continue to receive all your hair care from them?
5. When you experience a bad outcome from a harmful styling treatment, does the stylist try and deflect all blame back onto you?
6. Does your stylist regularly exceed recommended application times for permanent styling treatments such as chemical straightening and hair coloring?

If you answered yes to one or more of these questions, then you may need a new stylist. This is critically important for women with curly hair. Our hair is more fragile and can easily progress to a point of no return.

Now, don't think this is a reason to avoid stylists altogether; in fact, the message is quite the opposite.

The best stylists will tell you "no" when you ask for a chemical treatment or extensions while you are dealing with breakage. These types of treatments should really be performed when your hair is already healthy. They will also jump at the chance to teach you how to care for your hair between sessions so you continue to experience progress between appointments.

If your breakage is severe, I strongly recommend identifying a stylist at the beginning of your healthy hair journey. This is someone who should be honest with you about how much hair needs to be cut.

Stylists have access to hair products and appliances (like hair steamers and hooded dryers) that can enhance moisturization and may be too expensive for home use. Additionally, coupling your DIY hair care journey with a skilled stylist for the first three months can accelerate how quickly you see improvements.

Consider asking friends for recommendations and try out new stylists for minor services such as a wash and set. You'll likely be able to tell after one treatment if the stylist is one who thinks critically about hair. A great stylist prioritizes the long-term health of your hair over the short-term appearance. If you are not educated about what healthy hair practices are, a bad stylist may convince you that harmful styling habits are good for you.

To be clear, a great stylist is not one that simply makes you look good.

There are many stylists right now making a *fortune* because they have huge social media followings detailing the transformations of women with severe thinning and hair breakage. These pictures often start with a woman who has severe thinning and breakage and end with a woman with a new cut, color, and style (usually involving a very hot flat iron). Well, once the picture is over, the women are left with worsening breakage and damage, but the cameras are gone. That is *not* a great stylist.

A great stylist will come up with a long-term plan, perhaps spanning months to years, on how to nurture your hair back to health. You may not look Instagram ready immediately following your sessions but in the long run, your hair will thank you for it.

Twenty-Nine

Trim Your Split Ends Regularly

While long hair is not the goal for all women, I do realize that the goal for many women who read this book will be to grow their hair to longer lengths. Long hair comes with its own issues—specifically that it requires more maintenance than short hair. The most common mistake I see women making in their journey to long hair is refusing to cut off frayed, split ends.

It may sound counterintuitive, but if you want long hair, you have to get comfortable with cutting your hair. Split ends are the result of repetitive trauma to the hair. This leads to the loss of the outer portion of the hair, called the cuticle, which exposes the inner portion of the hair, the cortex. While conditioners can temporarily mend split ends, they cannot repair them completely, and over time, the split ends can travel up the hair and cause longer pieces of hair to break off. Things like chemical relaxers, hair color, and heat styling all increase the risk of getting split ends.

When you get regular trims, you can cut off the split ends before they travel up the hair shaft, thus minimizing the number of hairs that will be broken off at shorter lengths.

This leads to the inevitable question: *How often should I trim my hair?* Like almost everything in this book, it depends.

Hair grows at approximately half an inch per month, though this varies from person to person and differs even among people of different ethnic groups. Generally, hair grows a little faster in people of Asian descent and a little slower in people of African descent. If your hair grows pretty quickly and is unhealthy, you may need to trim split ends as often as every six to eight weeks. If your hair grows more slowly and/or it is well conditioned and healthy, you may only need to trim it every three to four months. If the point is to grow your hair, you certainly don't want to trim half an inch every six weeks, or it would take you years to grow your hair to your shoulders!

How much you trim mostly depends on how much damage you have. If you have not trimmed your hair in a year, you may need to lose a few inches needed to get you back on track. Generally, trimming off about one-fourth to half an inch every three months should do the trick. A more time-consuming but length-conserving method is to go strand by strand, snipping off only split ends. Typically, this is done more often so only small snips are needed. Over time, you may be able to conserve more length this way. Trims can be done at home with hair shears or with a trusted stylist. Trimming is the true definition of gaining by losing.

Thirty

Don't Be Afraid to Rock Your TWA

I remember the first time I, a curly 4C girl, visited a natural hair salon. The stylist, who was great, asked me what my goals were, and I told her, "To grow my hair as long as possible, ideally to my mid-back." This seemed like a reasonable goal, especially because I had been bombarded by images of "length checks" and "hair goals" on my social media, which implied that by simply going natural, I would achieve hair lengths like never before. She quickly brought me down to earth with a terse reply, "Long natural hair is much harder to take care of and grow than you think. You should consider wearing it short." I mean, wow, what a way to kill the mood! And what did she know anyway?

But of course, she was right. Growing long natural hair *is* hard, and short styles absolutely should be considered as it is easier to keep short hair healthy and moisturized. As I discussed in Chapter 4, there are evolutionary reasons tighter curl patterns are more prone to breakage after a certain length, but you should also know that type 4 curls are better suited to be worn short than any other curl pattern. In fact, type 4 hair is the only hair type that, when cut short, lays flat against the scalp in the correct orientation. Curly hair for the win!

So, while this book will certainly help you achieve your length goals, in case you are frustrated, I wanted to include a chapter on considering rocking your hair the exact way it's intended, as a teeny-weeny afro

(TWA). TWAs are low maintenance and keep the hair in its healthiest form. Moisturizing regularly will keep it hydrated and looking its best, and most importantly, short hair does not require lengthy styling sessions. If you are not sure if a TWA will look good on you, discuss it with your stylist. There are many ways to style TWAs that still create a very feminine appearance (if that is important to you). With these styles, you will also reap the benefits of transitioning to a healthy hair routine much sooner than 90 days.

Thirty-One

Let Your Curl Pattern and Density Guide Your Protective Styling Choices

Protective styles are considered a regular part of many curly girls' hair routines. The idea behind them is pretty straightforward—routine grooming, such as combing and brushing the hair regularly, can lead to breakage, so if the hair is tucked away, you can avoid this damage.

But the term 'protective styles' is really misleading for many women as these styles are often a significant cause of hair loss and breakage.

When I talk about protective styles, I am referring to most types of extensions (e.g., weaves, braids, or wigs) or any styles that use added hair. These protective styles can cause hair breakage in one of two ways:

1. Because extensions make it difficult to reach the hair (or, in the case of wigs, the hair is just braided and forgotten about), regular washing and conditioning of the hair do not occur. For those who are prone to having extremely dry hair, this is incredibly risky. This breakage can be accelerated during the takedown process (see Chapter 35).

2. These same protective styles can pull at the hairline and cause hair thinning, a condition called traction alopecia. Depending on your stage of traction alopecia, this can be very difficult to reverse (see Chapter 46).

Many people are familiar with thinning edges from protective styles but are not prepared for the severe breakage that happens from the hair drying out due to protective styles. This often happens when the style is removed and can be mistaken for shedding. In reality, the shed hair is often mixed in with broken hairs and it can be difficult to tell which is which. Having fistfuls of hair come out after taking down a braided style is never normal and should not be treated as such. If this is your typical experience and you've noticed that your hair growth seems stunted, you are likely breaking off your hair faster than it is growing.

Here are some styles that I generally recommend avoiding completely if you have ever experienced issues with hair breakage or thinning edges:

- Microbraids
- Sisterlocks (unless you have normal or high-density type 4 hair with NO prior hair loss issues—see Chapter 32)
- Glued in weaves
- Lace front wigs attached with glue or tape

There are, however, some less risky options, considering your curl pattern and hair density. Types 3A and 3B hair are fairly resistant to breakage, though styles may not last quite as long in these hair types as with hair types with tighter curl patterns. For these reasons, I will focus on types 3C–4C.

1. **3C/4A normal density hair:** Compared to other curl patterns, these curls are least likely to become dry, and as a result, least likely to experience breakage while in extensions. Additionally, women with this curl pattern are also less likely to experience thinning along the edges, especially with normal density hair. Consider these protective styles in moderation:

a. Box braids/Senegalese twists/jumbo braids, etc.
b. Sew-in weaves
c. Wigs
d. Crochet braids

2. **4A/4B normal density hair:** Though less likely to dry out than 4C hair, avoid styles that are kept in more than six weeks to avoid breakage. Wigs are fine if removed daily and hair is cleansed weekly. If you have low-density hair, avoid braided or sewn styles that can pull at the hairline (see Chapter 32 for styles to avoid). Consider these protective styles in moderation:

a. Box braids/Senegalese twists/jumbo braids, etc.
b. Sew-in weaves
c. Wigs (removed daily)
d. Locks (ideally greater than 5mm in width)
e. Crochet braids

3. **4C/4C+ normal density hair:** This hair type is the most likely to dry out and therefore is the most likely to be associated with significant shedding during the takedown process. Weaves, which nearly eliminate any ability to moisturize the hair should be avoided if possible. Because leave-in conditioner sprays can still moisturize the tips of the hair while in box braids, these are preferred to crochet braids if avoiding dry hair is a primary concern. However, crochet braids are associated with lower tension along the hairline, so depending on your area of concern, these may be a preferable choice. Consider low manipulation styles that do not involve synthetic hair instead (see Chapter 32 for recommendations).

a. Box braids/Senegalese twists/jumbo braids, etc.
b. Wigs (removed regularly/daily)
c. Locks (ideally greater than 5mm in width)

One parting word: If you have low-density 4C/4C+ plus hair, you will notice no recommendations for protective styles to consider. For those with low-density/fine hair in this curl pattern, you are unlikely to avoid damage in any protective style, so proceed with caution. It may be wise to avoid protective styles entirely.

Thirty-Two

Avoid Tight Hairstyles

S o now that you have figured out which styles are best for you, how can you ensure that you minimize your chances of hair loss?

When it comes to hair loss, one of the most vulnerable areas to lose hair is along the temples. It is here that most women notice hair thinning after pregnancy, as they age, and when wearing tight hairstyles. The first two cannot be avoided, but fortunately, the last one can. Tight hairstyles—including tight ponytails, braided extensions, weaves, dreadlocks, and wigs—all pull out the hair over time. While some women can wear beautifully braided hairstyles again and again with no issue, for most people this will lead to hair loss over time.

One of my favorite phrases is *"hair loss begets hair loss."* And what I mean by this is the exact styles that we use to cover up hair loss are often the same ones that make hair loss worse.

Braids can be an excellent way to camouflage hair loss, especially if the hair is parted correctly. I have seen very talented stylists figure out ways to attach braids to even the smallest patches of hair. This satisfies clients in the short run, but in the long run, these fragile patches are easily pulled out and hair loss gets worse . . . quickly.

Wigs are notorious for pulling out hair along the hairline, especially when they are glued in place, but can also cause hair loss for a variety of reasons (see Chapters 33, 34).

Over time, **dreadlocks** can also pull out the hairline, especially when they are retwisted on a regular basis. While this keeps them looking "neat," the damage can be swift and unrelenting. Additionally, as the hair grows and sheds hairs and new growth is incorporated into the lock, the weight of the lock adds additional tension to the hairline as well as other parts of the scalp. Taken together, these issues can cause women to suddenly wake up one day and notice their hairline has moved way back. Since locks carry a spiritual meaning for many, cutting them can be a very emotional process.

Sisterlocks cause more damage than regular locks because each lock uses only a few hairs to hold the entire weight of the lock. As the hair grows and becomes heavier, this tension causes these small hairs to snap quickly. Over time, this hair loss can become permanent. In essence, sisterlocks are the dreadlock equivalent of microbraids. They are best reserved for those with high-density, resilient hair in women with no evidence of thinning along the hairline. These are the women that I have seen tolerate them best without issue.

In my clinic, I see several patients with hair loss from sisterlocks, and it can be very difficult to reverse. I also have many patients who have thinning and breakage, and in wanting to remain natural, they feel like sisterlocks are a safe alternative. This is truly not the case. On the bright side, I have seen many women reverse worsening hair loss simply by cutting their sisterlocks, though this is a decision that isn't to be taken lightly as locks are often considered to have a spiritual connection as well. While I would never encourage someone with sisterlocks to cut their hair if they are experiencing no issues, I think it is prudent to think twice about installing them if you have already noticed thinning. If you have sisterlocks in place and have only noticed thinning as they grow longer, it is possible that cutting your locks to shoulder length and decreasing your touch-up frequency may also help minimize breakage.

If you are used to wearing one of these styles and have not experienced hair loss (or you have, and it's just a little bit), then that is great.

Early on, hair loss from tightly braided styles is reversible and will grow back with just a little TLC. For other women, however, the hair loss can be severe and permanent (see Chapter 45). At this stage, often the only thing that will grow the hair back is a hair transplant, and those cost anywhere between $10k–$30k. Ask yourself, are your extensions really worth that? While you are reading this book and focusing on improving the strength and length of your hair, do not forget about your hairline. Here are some easy tips you can follow to minimize stress in this sensitive area:

1. Avoid applying extensions to hair that has been recently chemically straightened. Chemically straightened hair is already weakened, so it makes sense that adding extensions increases the chances of hair loss.
2. Consider extensions that apply less tension to your hairline, like a faux bun or ponytail.
3. Use best practices while wearing a wig (see Chapters 33, 34)
4. If you wear dreadlocks, extend the time between touch-up sessions so that you are retwisting less often.
5. Before adding weaved extensions, braid cornrows in a horizontal or circular direction around the scalp, instead of vertically from front to back, to minimize pulling the hair backward, away from the hairline.

Thirty-Three

Beware Hair Loss from Wig Use

In the world of hair care, there is likely no double-edged sword like the wig. Wigs are great for several reasons: they allow you to change your appearance quickly, they're chic, natural-looking, and obviously way more low maintenance than styling your own hair.

But let's focus on that last part. I cannot tell you how many women I have met who are natural but are so overwhelmed by taking care of natural hair that they resort to only wearing wigs. Many women choose wigs because they believe they are less likely to cause damage to the hairline like braids and weaves. This creates a false sense of security that wigs are a safe alternative to other forms of extensions, but this is not necessarily true.

Remember, natural hair only thrives when it is taken care of in the right way. That means weekly deep conditioning, moisturizing with a leave-in conditioner multiple times a week, and sealing with an oil.

Unfortunately, wigs can wick away a lot of moisture from the hair, and keeping the hair braided down for weeks or even months at a time can lead to severe matting. A busy lifestyle means that this can happen before you even realize it. In fact, the worst cases of hair breakage that I come across in my clinic are almost always in women who wear wigs daily.

Furthermore, wigs are a common cause of traction alopecia as they can pull the hair on your hairline over time. The constant friction can wreak havoc on the very fragile hairs dotting your hairline. Over time, this hair loss can be irreversible.

I recognize the difficulty in leading a very busy lifestyle while also trying to keep your hair healthy. If you love wigs and would still like to incorporate them occasionally, here is what I recommend:

1. **Limit yourself to wigs that you can remove every night.** Wigs that stay in place for days and weeks at a time can worsen breakage and hair loss.

2. **Use a satin or silk wig cap to prevent dryness of the hair.** This is especially important for women with type 4 since dryness can be a major cause of breakage. Wearing a wig without a cap or with a polyester cap will increase the dryness experienced and render your deep conditioner less effective

3. **Use a leave-in conditioner regularly to make sure your hair stays moisturized during the week.**

4. **If you have cornrows underneath your braids, unbraid them weekly before washing.** Cornrows and other braids tuck in your ends, which need to be moisturized during wash sessions. Make sure you are thoroughly cleansing and moisturizing your hair if you wear a wig.

5. **Find hairstyles that you are comfortable with that will allow you to limit your wig to occasional use.** Even if you do everything right, wearing a wig almost daily will still cause damage, so the less often you can wear them, the better.

Thirty-Four

Just say "No!" to Wig Glues and Adhesives

S o, back when only grandmothers wore wigs, they were designed to be worn for a few hours at a time. As a result, most wigs simply came with comb attachments or clips to keep them in place for a short time.

Fast forward to the present day, and wigs are arguably the most popular styling choice among women, including celebrities. When celebrities wear wigs, they are able to switch between many different styles in a matter of minutes. Lace front wigs are particularly popular because they create a seamless transition between the wig and the hairline, making them look very authentic.

However, given the difficulty with applying lace fronts correctly, it is no surprise that many women prefer to apply the wig once and have it stay in place for weeks at a time. This is done using very effective glues, sprays, and adhesives.

I recognize that given their popularity, many of you reading this chapter may have become quite accustomed to wearing wigs daily, but my goal is not to make you feel bad! If you are reading this and you have fallen victim to a heavy rotation of adhesives and glues, know that there are safer ways to apply wigs but it is also important that you do not miss the big point:

No matter how careful you are with the use of wig glues, regular use of any adhesive on the hairline will eventually pull your hair out.

Of course, if you have a very thick hairline and only wear wigs occasionally, this is not a huge deal. But if you have resorted to wearing wigs as your go-to hairstyle and are already noticing thinning, this problem will worsen over time.

In Chapter 45, I will talk about traction alopecia, but you should know that even a single use of an adhesive can take you from a thinning hairline that just needs a little help to complete baldness in that area that only improves with a surgical hair transplant.

Glues and tapes cause issues for multiple reasons:

1. **Glues and tapes can pull out small hairs along the hairline with each use, even if removed properly.** Even with the best dissolving agents or oils, it is impossible to eliminate this hair loss, and over time, the loss adds up and quickly becomes severe

2. **Many people are allergic to the active ingredients in glues and tapes, leading to a severe allergic reaction, even if you have used them before.** The active ingredients in many adhesives are called *acrylates*. Realize, the skin has to be exposed to an allergen at least once before a reaction develops. This means that you could be using your favorite glue for years and one day it goes rogue on you and leads to severe scalp inflammation. When this happens, hair loss is often drastic . . . and permanent. Oftentimes, severe reactions require oral medications to treat, while mild reactions may improve with over-the-counter treatments.

To help decrease your reliance on adhesives to place your wig, consider these tips:

1. **Try and become more comfortable with removing your wig nightly.** This means that you will rely more heavily on applying wigs using comb attachments and bobby pins. While this can still cause some traction alopecia, it is not as dangerous as adhesives and glues.

2. **If you can't quit adhesives cold turkey, start with adhesives that are less bonding.** If you are using thick layers of glue, first try to move to adhesives tapes, then eventually to comb attachments. Every little bit counts.

The unfortunate truth is, it is hard to get the wig security that heavy glues provide through other means, so eventually, you may have to be okay with alternatives that make your wig feel less secure. If you have already noticed gradual hair thinning from your wigs, consider eliminating wig use altogether and review Chapters 45 and 46 to see if you can work on thickening these areas as soon as possible.

Thirty-Five

Take the Time to Detangle Your Hair When Removing Protective Styles

Talk about a hair-saving tip! I'm sure many of you reading this book have experienced this scenario. Picture this:

You have a trip to Jamaica planned and cannot wait to enjoy some water activities. While you rarely wear extensions, you decide to install a cute set of box braids. You plan to leave them in for four weeks, but when you return from vacation, you realize that work has become even busier. Given the ease of wearing the braids, you decide to keep them in longer. Initially just for eight weeks, but before you know it, twelve weeks have passed, and your scalp is starting to get very itchy. You plan for a marathon braid removal session and have an appointment with your stylist in the morning. After six hours, your braids are out but they are heavily matted. You spend 15 minutes detangling but realize that time is limited, so you leave the rest for the next day. The only problem is, your stylist does not have the time to detangle your hair either, so after a painful ten minutes of combing your hair out, you proceed to get it washed. This washing only worsens the matting, and your stylist delivers the bad news: your hair cannot be salvaged and must be cut.

Ouch. Talk about a nightmare. While some of the details may be different, this scenario is all too common and can lead to severe hair loss.

As I've mentioned earlier, curly hair is prone to breakage, partially because tangling is so common. These tangles can lead to massive hair breakage if not approached carefully. For this reason, careful detangling after wash sessions is critically important. But this pales in comparison to the need to detangle after wearing protective styles. Curly hair becomes easily matted and sticks together as dirt, skin cells, and other debris get trapped within the braids. The longer a hairstyle is worn, the more significant the matting. If hair is washed before the hair is detangled, it is not unusual for the entire hair to become tangled into a nest-like mess. This can lead to fistfuls of hair loss in a single sitting.

So how can you avoid this? Here are some tips:

1. As an oversimplified rule of thumb, set aside one to two hours of detangling for every month that the protective style is in place. So, in the example above, our curly-haired sister should have expected to spend *at least* three hours detangling. You can expect to spend less time if you have type 3 curls and more time if you are type 4C.
2. Avoid time-sensitive deadlines that put pressure on you to detangle quickly. For example, if you are expecting to detangle for three hours, don't simply block out 4:00–7:00 p.m. with a 7:30 p.m. dinner scheduled. Plan to set aside the whole day so you can institute breaks as needed.
3. Condition your hair overnight *before* you detangle the next day. In fact, the greenhouse treatment (see Chapter 22) is perfect for this. This can easily cut down your detangling time in half as it softens the matting on the hair.

Thirty-Six

Incorporate Apple Cider Vinegar Rinses While Wearing Protective Styles

By now we have gone through all of the dos and don'ts of protective styles and you have hopefully figured out which styles are most compatible with your hair type. So, what else can you do to ensure you don't have a setback while wearing your protective style?

Well, if you are in a style that allows you to access your scalp easily—like box braids, crochet braids, Senegalese twists, etc.—the best thing you can do is try to continue your wash routine as best as possible. This means weekly cleansing and regular use of a leave-in conditioner.

However, typical shampoos and conditioners can be very difficult to completely rinse out of the hair and can also mess up your hairstyle.

Well, apple cider vinegar is an excellent option. Apple cider vinegar is acidic, meaning, it leaves a positive charge on the hair. This positive charge leaves the hair feeling soft and manageable, all while doing a great job of cleansing the scalp. You can make your own diluted preparations or use preprepared rinses that have a mild lather (see Appendix B for product recommendations).

After cleansing, you can go straight to applying a leave-in conditioner spray followed by a light oil. Repeat this once every one or two weeks while in your protective style to minimize dryness as well as breakage.

Thirty-Seven

For Type 3 Hair: Embrace Wash and Go

One of the core tenets of maintaining healthy natural hair is to avoid over-manipulation of the hair. This can come in the form of frequent use of combs and brushes or simply frequent styling like twist-outs or braid-outs. Frequent manipulation of the hair can lead to easy breakage, and this idea is one of the reasons that protective styles are so popular. Low manipulation styles, on the other hand, are styles that need minimal upkeep, and ideally, can last from one washing session to the next and are achieved without the use of added hair.

One style that is an excellent option for type 3 (and 4A) curls is a style called a "wash and go." This style takes advantage of well-moisturized, defined curls that occur on freshly washed hair by keeping them in place for a week or longer. This is the perfect style to take you from wash day to wash day. Because this style is easiest to achieve in well-defined curl patterns, it is ideal for types 3A–4A curl patterns. Women with 4C hair should NOT rely on wash-and-go styles because infrequent moisturizing (i.e., only applying leave-in conditioner on wash day) while wearing the hair loosely can lead to severe tangling, and ultimately, breakage. Instead, women with 4C hair can achieve similar results with twist-outs and braid-outs, which allow moisture to set in a braided style for a few days before the hair is worn loosely.

So how do you achieve a wash and go?

1. Start by washing and deep conditioning your hair.
2. Follow with an intense rinse-out conditioner (don't be afraid to add a little extra).
3. While the hair is still wet, begin to run your favorite leave-in cream and/or styling gel through individual strands of hair. Depending on your density, this may take up to an hour or more to do. The more you focus on hydrating each strand, the more defined your final style will be.
4. Dry your hair. This can be done overnight, but many women prefer to use a diffuser, a type of blow-dryer that spreads heat evenly over the hair and maximizes volume without disrupting the curls, to help speed up the process.

These steps are pretty non-specific and vary by curl type. If you have a looser 3A–3B curl pattern with low-density hair, avoid thick creams, which may feel too heavy. You may be better off using a light styling lotion followed by a gel, or curling creams. Alternatively, if you are a type 4A, you may have to use two or more products to achieve a well-defined curl.

Thirty-Eight

Use a Lye Relaxer Only

P eople often assume that because I am a dermatologist specializing in hair loss, I am an enemy of chemical relaxers. Many of my patients who relax their hair will start their appointments defiantly proclaiming that they refuse to stop relaxing their hair because that is what they are used to dermatologists telling them to do. So, let me start out by saying this:

I am not an enemy of chemical relaxers,
but my goal is to make my patients more
knowledgeable about the side effects.

I am not an enemy of relaxers because I know there are several pros associated with the use of relaxers, such as:

- Ease of styling (this is huge and can mean the difference between minutes in the mirror versus hours!)
- Permanent straightening for those who like to wear their hair straight most of the time
- General personal preference

Of course, as a hair loss specialist, these days I concern myself more with the cons of relaxers as I think it is prudent for each person to balance the pros and cons in their life before proceeding with any hairstyling choice. These include:

- Chemical burns
- Temporary or permanent hair loss
- Recurrent hair breakage

To understand the ways by which relaxers can lead to hair loss, we should start with the basics.

WHAT IS A CHEMICAL RELAXER?

Chemical relaxers are most commonly divided into lye and no-lye formulations. Lye formulations are typically available only in salons and contain sodium hydroxide. No-lye formulations, on the other hand, are available over the counter and often must be mixed prior to use. The most popular formulations contain calcium hydroxide (base) and guanidine carbonate (activator), which when mixed together form guanidine hydroxide.

If you recall from your high school chemistry class, pH scales run between 1–14, with numbers below 7 representing acids and numbers above 7 representing bases. Products containing pH levels at the extreme ends of the scale contain ingredients that can easily burn through skin, plastic, and even metal, depending on the concentration. Lye formulations typically measure at a pH of 11-13 and no-lye formulations typically measure at a pH of 9–11. Therefore, people generally associate lye relaxers with more severe burns than no-lye formulations. Ironically, the use of a lye formulation and its associated burning sensation makes it *less likely* to overprocess the hair. This is because users are less likely to leave the relaxer on longer than recommended. Overprocessing is a primary cause of breakage and sudden hair shedding that many people associate with relaxer use, but overprocessing is more likely to occur with the use of at-home no-lye relaxers. Keep reading below to find out why.

WHY ARE LYE RELAXERS BETTER THAN NO-LYE RELAXERS?

I know the idea that lye relaxers are preferred to no-lye relaxers may sound crazy to some. For women like me who have been familiar with relaxers their whole lives, no-lye relaxers are considered the safe version of relaxers because they do not burn the scalp. This is true; no-lye relaxers, available over the counter, are sold directly to consumers because they are less likely to burn the scalp. However, no-lye relaxers contain calcium hydroxide (the white stuff in the jar), which, when combined with guanidine carbonate (the liquid stuff in the bottle), forms guanidine hydroxide with calcium carbonate as a by-product. Have you ever heard of limestone? Yeah, that's calcium carbonate. Ever heard of limewater or builder's lime? That's calcium hydroxide. While these no-lye relaxers are effective at relaxing the hair, these calcified deposits build up on the hair over time, causing it to become dull and more susceptible to damage. That dullness is one of the reasons why hair that is relaxed at home does not look quite as shiny as hair that has been consistently relaxed in a salon.

But there is another reason I prefer salon relaxers: the burn. You read that right. While I never advise that relaxer is kept on the hair until the scalp burns, the mere fear of burning the scalp because of the caustic characteristics of lye relaxers means that it is rarely left on longer than instructed. These are different from home relaxers, which users frequently leave on for much longer than instructed in hopes of getting hair that is "bone straight." Many of us, including myself, are guilty of this bad habit. Instead of relying on a timer to estimate when the processing of the hair is complete, a tingling and/or a mild burning sensation is often considered a more "reliable" metric that women use to inform them of when to rinse relaxer from the hair.

But make no mistake: *Burning and tingling sensations are a sign that the skin is getting irritated, not that the relaxer is working.*

Because no-lye relaxers are designed to lessen the risk of skin irritation, they are often left on longer than lye-containing relaxer formulations.

This means that women are much more likely to overprocess their hair using no-lye relaxer kits. This leads to more breakage, more dulling, and generally, more problems.

The decision to relax the hair should never be taken lightly. It is a permanent, irreversible treatment that works by first weakening your hair strands. If your desire is to have hair that is thick and dense, a relaxer will likely do the opposite. However, it is a wiser alternative than using extreme heat every week to straighten the hair.

Here are some tips for minimizing damage from relaxers:

1. If you want to truly just "relax" your curls and not get it bone straight, consider asking your stylist to apply relaxers with a lower concentration of sodium hydroxide. These relaxers are typically marketed to kids or have the words "mild" on the box. While this will not eliminate the damage experienced from using a relaxer, it may minimize it.
2. Use a lye relaxer only and make sure it is applied by a stylist.
3. Get a hydrating or deep conditioner treatment applied the same day as your relaxer.
4. Apply a protein treatment to your hair weekly (but not on the day of your relaxer) to prevent further breakage.
5. Deep condition your hair every time you wash.
6. Eliminate or limit the use of heat styling tools to straighten your hair.

Incorporating these tips will not only work to minimize damage, but for some, may improve length retention in the long run.

Thirty-Nine

Space Out Chemical Styling Treatments

The great thing about hair is that it's always growing. Sometimes, the worst thing about hair is that it's always growing. Ugh! This becomes an issue when you're a big fan of permanent styling treatments like relaxers and hair coloring. That's because, every few weeks, like clockwork, you realize that you're due for another treatment.

While it may be tempting to stack these treatments closely together to avoid messing up your style, it is actually very important to make sure your treatments are spaced far apart. On average, hair grows about half an inch per month, sometimes more, sometimes less. It's much harder to limit the application of relaxer or hair color to a small half-inch strip of hair than it is to limit it to a one-and-a-half-inch strip. Getting frequent touch-ups increases the risk that hair that has already been treated is accidentally treated twice, thus doubling the damage. If accidental overtreatment is unavoidable, spacing out treatments also gives you more opportunity to strengthen your hair between touch-ups with protein treatments and deep conditioning.

Certainly, all of this may be much easier said than done, but it's yet another simple tweak to your hair care regimen that could pay dividends in the long run.

Forty

Want Straight Hair but Not Ready for a Full-Strength Relaxer? Try a Texturizer

The first thing you should know before reading this chapter is that *texturizer ingredients are identical to relaxer ingredients, just in a much lower strength.*

Texturizers are the source of the original "Jheri curl" hairstyle. Instead of straightening the curl completely like a typical relaxer, it slightly loosens the curl pattern. If you have a really tight curl pattern (like 4C or 4C+), with a texturizer treatment your hair will still likely look "natural," but with a curl pattern that is more similar to 4A or 4B hair. However, there will be subtle differences as your hair will look slightly different compared to someone who is a "true" 4A or 4B, and may not hold twist-out and braid-out styles in the same way. Another potential downside is that if you truly desire straight hair but opt for a texturizer instead of a relaxer, you will likely still notice your hair revert to a curly pattern when it's humid and it will never quite take on a sleek, straight appearance.

But there are many reasons to consider texturizing type 4 hair. For instance, because texturizing the hair will make it more porous, meaning it is more open to accepting moisture, it will be easier to moisturize the hair during deep conditioning sessions. This is really helpful for women who struggle with this issue. If dry hair and difficulty retaining moisture are your primary reasons for hair breakage, you may notice an *increase* in length retention by moving to a texturizer. You will also notice that once the hair is texturized, styling time will be cut down as well.

So how should you proceed if you are interested in trying out a texturizer treatment?

1. **A texturizer should be applied by a stylist only.** This is to ensure consistent application throughout and minimize the likelihood of scalp burning or hair loss.
2. **Use a lye-only texturizer.** This means that the active ingredient in this case is typically sodium hydroxide. If the texturizer has to be mixed before applying it to the hair, this means that it is a no-lye product.
3. **Keep your hair moisturized as much as possible to minimize breakage**. This means incorporating regular deep conditioning treatments and leave-in conditioners throughout the week.
4. **Don't overestimate the level of straightening you will achieve.** Some women opt for a texturizer when they actually want to be relaxed. This can lead to an over-reliance on heat straightening tools, which subsequently leads to severe breakage. Be realistic about the type of hairstyles that will be feasible with a texturizer.
5. **Space out texturizer sessions.** Even though texturizers do not straighten the hair as much as a relaxer, it does not mean that a texturizer can be applied more often. Overapplication can lead to breakage, just as it would with a relaxer.

Texturizers can be helpful to decrease styling time, and if you're experiencing significant dryness leading to breakage, you may notice an overall improvement in length retention and hair health. Just remember, a texturizer is a permanent treatment, so once you make the decision to texturize, plan to stick with it.

Forty-One

Cut Back on Heat Styling

I am going to go out on a limb and guess that almost every person reading this book owns either a blow-dryer, flat iron, or both. These tools continue to be some of the most popular hair styling tools regardless of hair type. These heat styling tools have evolved over the past few decades, and now it's easy to find blow-dryers and flat irons that promise to eliminate all damage and even make your hair *healthier.*

Well, I will tell you right now that that is false. But one of the upsides of flat ironing the hair straight is that it allows all the hair to lie in one direction. This allows light to hit in a way that boosts shine, an effect that is further enhanced after the use of hair serums. As most of us know, the shine is short-lived and gone by the next day and is not to be mistaken as a surrogate sign of health.

Flat-ironing takes advantage of the hair shafts' ability to temporarily change shape using the hair's hydrogen bonds. Applying water (i.e. H_2O) to the hair restores the hydrogen bonds and returns the hair to its natural wavy or curly state. However, healthy hair burns at 451.4 degrees Fahrenheit and damaged hair burns at much lower temperatures. Once the hair burns, the damage is irreversible, and it cannot be restored to health. Even if your hair is not completely burned from one treatment, heat styling does damage the hair, and that damage continues to add up each time heat is used. This is because each time the hair is exposed to heat, water is rapidly pushed out of the hair, and in the process, leaves holes in the hair that leave it fragile and more prone to damage.

So, what should you do if just can't find a way to give up on heat? Try these adjustments

1. **Consider air-drying your hair for as long as possible before blow-drying (see Chapter 17).** The less water that is pushed out of the hair by a blow-dryer, the less damage you will experience. Wait until your hair is at least 75–80 percent dry before reaching for your blow-dryer.

2. **Try a ceramic or titanium-coated flat iron, which can lessen damage during flat-ironing by minimizing friction between the heat tool and hair strand.**

3. **Cut the number of times you blow-dry and flat-iron your hair as much as you can.** If you are experiencing a lot of breakage, then using heat on a regular basis won't cut it. Consider cutting back on your heat styling by half and eventually decreasing use to a couple of times a month at most.

4. **Use a heat protectant every time you use heat.** These products help decrease the amount of heat transferred to the hair during the straightening process.

5. **Set your flat iron to 350 degrees or less.**

6. **Deep condition your hair before every flat-ironing session**. As we have discussed, dry hair is more prone to damage. Flat-ironing dry hair is kind of like starting a flame in a dry, California forest; you should expect a burn. Treating your hair to an intense moisturizing session allows it to withstand more heat and thereby minimize damage.

7. **Blow-dry your hair on a cool setting.** You can do this by pulling the hair taut while blow-drying on cool air and still get the hair pretty straight, with much less damage.

8. **If you prefer to wear your hair straight most of the time, choose a permanent straightener, such as a chemical relaxer**

or other straightening treatments, instead. These treatments are designed to chemically alter the pattern of your hair, so you won't have to straighten your hair artificially on a daily basis (see Chapters 38, 40). In the end, the damage you experience from these treatments will likely be less than the damage from daily blow-drying and flat-ironing your hair.

If all of this fails and you continue to experience breakage and split ends from using heat, then listen to your hair and drop heat for good. Some people, especially those with thin, fine hair, may just not be able to withstand the damage associated with heat. And you know what they say to do if you can't stand the heat . . .

Forty-Two

Sleep on a Satin Pillowcase at Night to Curb Hair Breakage

Ever woken up to broken hairs on your pillowcase? I know I have. By this point in the book, you have seen me go on and on about the importance of keeping your hair well hydrated and moisturized. Well, most pillowcases, especially those made of cotton, help achieve just the opposite. This is because cotton does a great job of wicking moisture away from surfaces and has a rougher texture than satin or silk. Ever been splashed in a cotton shirt? It dries pretty quickly. Get splashed in a satin shirt, and you'll feel soaked for hours. Additionally, the constant friction from tossing and turning on a cotton surface can be enough to break fragile hair strands. Switching to a satin or silk pillowcase will minimize the breakage you experience overnight by lowering the amount of friction experienced. Similarly, wearing a silk or satin headscarf or cap at night will have the same effect and help preserve hairstyles overnight.

While this may seem like a minor adjustment, sleeping with a satin cap or pillowcase can be a game changer for those with curly hair. You can easily find satin-lined caps at beauty supply stores and satin pillowcases for purchase online.

Forty-Three

Essential Oils Are for the Scalp, Not the Hair

One of the important things to know early on is the role of oils when it comes to hair and scalp health. There are two main groups of oils: essential oils and carrier oils.

Essential oils include oils like peppermint, rosemary, thyme, oregano, etc. There is a fair amount of evidence that suggests that essential oils can be used to treat inflammation on the scalp, such as scalp flaking. And though some people believe they may help with hair growth, the data is more limited here. When using essential oils, very specific blends are often suggested, though there are some essential oils that can be used alone and simply mixed with a carrier oil (see Chapter 45 for an oil mixture to try).

But you should think of essential oils as medicine, in that they are thought to have biological activity. For this reason, essential oils are only meant to be applied to the scalp. It's important to remember that the scalp is just skin, and is living, but the hair is not living (for example, when a hair strand breaks, you feel no pain). You cannot exert a medicinal action on something that is not living.

Another thing to remember is that because essential oils are, in essence, medicinal, they too can carry some side effects. Even herbal remedies can be risky, and you should do your due diligence before deciding which essential oils to try (see Appendix C). Some examples of reported side effects to essential oils are listed below:

Pregnancy Complications	Associated with Seizures	Can Mimic Estrogen Activity	Associated with Respiratory Issues in Babies	Can Cause Skin Irritation
Peppermint	Eucalyptus	Lavender	Eucalyptus	Tea Tree
Rosemary	Camphor	Tea Tree	Peppermint	
Camphor				
Thyme				

Carrier oils, on the other hand, include oils like avocado, grapeseed, olive oils, etc. These are not assumed to have any medicinal properties but are primarily used for purposes such as cooking and moisturizing the skin and hair. In fact, one of their other purposes is to dilute essential oils, which should never be applied directly to the skin in their pure form due to the chance of irritation. Check out Chapter 23 for suggestions on how to apply carrier oils to the hair and keep reading to find out my favorite essential oil mixture.

Forty-Four

Try an Essential Oil Blend for Hair Growth

A s I have mentioned in Chapter 43, there are few scientific studies that suggest that essential oils can lead to hair growth. One of the few exceptions is a study supporting the use of an essential oil blend consisting of cedarwood, thyme, lavender, and rosemary oil diluted in a carrier oil mix containing jojoba and grapeseed oil. In this study, doctors focused on patients with a specific type of hair loss called alopecia areata. In this autoimmune condition, the body's cells, designed to attack bacteria and viruses, instead begin to attack the hair follicles leading to coin-shaped patches on the scalp. In this study, half of the patients with alopecia areata were treated with the essential oil blend and the other half were treated with a placebo consisting of just the grapeseed and jojoba oil. After seven months, they noticed more patients treated with the essential oil blend (44 percent) had at least some hair growth compared to those who used the placebo blend (6 percent) (see Appendix C for more information).

Even though essential oils are available at any vitamin store, they can still cause severe allergic reactions, especially if not diluted first with inactive/carrier oils. Before you start, apply the combination oil behind your ear to see if you react. If you notice a reaction, then this may not be for you. Also, in general, they should be avoided by women who are pregnant, have high blood pressure, or have a history of seizures (see Chapter

44). If you're interested in trying this blend for thinning areas (after you have received approval from your doctor first!), then you can try the same dilution used in the study:

- 2 drops thyme oil
- 3 drops lavender oil
- 3 drops rosemary oil
- 2 drops cedarwood oil
- 3 mL jojoba oil
- 20 mL grapeseed oil

Combine all the oils as listed above into one container. Massage three drops into thinning areas for two minutes. Cover with a warm towel afterward for 10–15 minutes. Repeat every night. As with all things regarding hair, this method requires patience—the ingredients can be tough to find, and it may take months to see hair growth. All that aside, if you are a fan of essential oils, this may be worth a try.

Forty-Five

Address Your Traction Alopecia

I n Chapter 32, I discussed several styles to avoid that can gradually thin out your hairline. But if you're reading this book, there is a chance that you may have already noticed some gradual thinning of your edges over time. The medical term for this is "traction alopecia."

Traction alopecia is a medical condition that causes women to lose hair along their frontal hairline. This is especially common in women with tightly curled hair by nature of the tension created by some of the most popular styles. Many of the styles deemed "protective" can often lead to irreversible damage.

You have already gone through the process of determining whether or not you should be incorporating protective styles in your routine in Chapter 31. Once you have noticed that your hairline is thinning, the next step is identifying your stage of traction alopecia. When I evaluate patients with traction alopecia, I typically divide its severity into one of three stages. Understanding the severity of your disease will dictate what styles and treatments you are eligible for:

Stage 1: Wearing extensions by choice. In this stage, you may notice subtle thinning of your hairline, but your hair bounces back once you integrate breaks between styles. No medical treatment is required at this stage, and even minor interventions like massaging the scalp may encourage regrowth. _Recommended extensions frequency: Maximum two to three times a year (for a maximum of 6-8 weeks at a time)_

Stage 2: **You notice your edges have thinned . . . by a lot.** The thinning may have happened so slowly over the years that it has taken a while for you to even realize it. You realize (or are told by your dermatologist) that you must lay off extensions indefinitely, perhaps forever, if you want to maintain what you have. Medical treatment, like minoxidil, is used to rescue dormant follicles and improve density but must be continued forever to maintain progress. At this stage, the follicles have been so injured that they require constant medical therapy to produce normal hair. _Recommended extensions frequency: Zero to one time per year (six to eight weeks at a time) limited to special occasions only._

Stage 3: Sadly, this is the point of no return. At this point, your edges have thinned out so severely that you notice much of your hairline is now smooth bald. Sometimes it is hard to identify the cause because for several years prior to this point (when you were in stage 1 or 2), you made sure to wear extensions that didn't feel "tight." Unfortunately, for many women in stage 2 or stage 3 traction alopecia, extensions do not have to feel tight to pull out the hair. In stage 3, you are no longer wearing extensions by choice, but you have now found yourself in a position where you HAVE to wear extensions just to cover your area of hair loss. At this stage, medical treatments like minoxidil are unlikely to be effective and the only treatment is surgical hair transplant. This is an excellent option . . . if you can afford it. It typically costs $10,000–$20,000. However, once the transplant is completed, the hair restoration is permanent (as long as it is not pulled out by extensions again). _Recommended extensions frequency: If unable to afford a hair transplant, you can wear extensions as often as needed to feel comfortable with your appearance. At this stage, taking breaks will not lead to hair regrowth, so feeling comfortable in your skin is the best approach! Post-hair transplant—zero to one time per year._

Many women would rather be told they have a life-threatening condition causing hair loss than hear that their extensions have led to hair loss. I get it. There was a time in my life when I only felt "presentable" with weaves or braids, and this is still the case for many. I find myself having this tough conversation at least once a day, and it doesn't get easier. I work hard to save the women in stage 2. However, it is so important to embrace your hair and feel comfortable wearing your hair as often as possible to minimize permanent hair loss. It is my hope that this book will help you feel comfortable doing that.

Forty-Six

Grow Your Edges Back
with Minoxidil

O h, minoxidil! When it comes to hair growth treatments, minoxidil may have the worst PR agent out there, but it is honestly a dermatologist's best friend.

Minoxidil is the only FDA-approved topical treatment for hair loss and is available over the counter without a prescription. Though it is mostly marketed to treat male and female pattern thinning, I find myself using it most often for my patients to treat traction alopecia. Success rates with minoxidil are quite high, estimated to be between 60–80 percent (compare this to essential oils which are likely more in the 5 percent success range).

As I mentioned in the last chapter, stage 2 disease is the stage of disease that is most suitable for medical therapy. At this stage, avoiding tight hairstyles and massaging with a scalp oil are simply not enough to regrow the edges. If you have been stuck in stage 2 for years, this is probably something you have recognized deep down.

Many women don't like the idea of using minoxidil because they have heard that once you use it, you cannot stop using it or everything you have grown will fall out.

This is *true*.

But this is no different than any other product applied to the skin. Think about having extremely dry skin. If a friend recommends a moisturizer that will make your skin look brand-new, it is already assumed that you have to use that product forever to sustain results. If you just use it for two weeks and stop using lotion again, then guess what? Your skin will still be extremely dry. That does not mean that the lotion didn't work, it just means that the benefits are transient.

To put it another way, think of minoxidil like watering a plant. Let's say you are consistent about watering a plant every day for six months, then suddenly you're whisked away to Paris and can't water it for two months. Well, when you return, the plant will likely be dead. Certainly, you won't think that the water killed the plant; you will realize that the plant needs consistent, uninterrupted nurturing to thrive.

If it seems like I am dragging the idea of committing to minoxidil long term, it's because I am. The biggest hurdle to using minoxidil is staying on minoxidil, despite its effectiveness. But it is actually the most effective treatment for traction alopecia that exists.

Interested in starting minoxidil and have the go-ahead from your doctor? Here are my suggestions:

1. **Opt for the solution formulation as opposed to the foam.** The foam is great for people with straight hair who wash their hair daily, but if you have curly hair, the foam will build up quickly since you are only washing every one or two weeks.
2. **Follow the application of the solution with a light oil every time.** The solution dries very easily (this is great, no build-up!), but this can also cause the scalp to become very dry and itchy. Apply your favorite carrier oil with each application (see Chapter 23 for suggestions).
3. **Limit application to your hairline only.** Minoxidil only works if it is directly applied to the scalp, which is quite easy to do along the hairline. If you apply the solution to areas where there is a lot more hair (like the central scalp), you are likely to experience breakage in areas where it is applied because of its drying properties.

4. **Be patient.** Minoxidil takes a minimum of three months to work and up to six months before you can notice a difference. I have had many patients stop using it after two weeks because it "didn't work." I think this expectation of rapid results is partially created by false marketing from companies who insist that hair growth can occur in a matter of days. If your traction alopecia has reached stage 2, you have likely already tried treatments that have not been effective, so consider minoxidil worth the wait.

5. **If you notice irritation, stop using it!** As I said above, minoxidil can dry out the scalp, and certain people are more sensitive than others to this reaction. Please do not continue using it if you are noticing itching or pain of any kind.

6. **If you notice no improvement after six months, consult a dermatologist.** In my previous book, I use the three-month mark, and the reality is, there is often noticeable improvement by then. However, I have realized that when you are looking at your scalp in the mirror every day, even obvious improvements can seem subtle. Six months makes it more likely that you will notice the benefits if it is working. That being said, there are many forms of hair loss that affect the hairline, some of which will not respond to minoxidil at all, and a dermatologist is needed to provide an accurate diagnosis. Additionally, dermatologists have access to prescription treatments that may be effective for patients who have not responded to over-the-counter therapy.

Forty-Seven

Make sure to Address
Your Dandruff

Dandruff, also called seborrheic dermatitis, is a very common scalp condition. Many people notice scalp flaking and think their scalp must be dry, but this is actually a myth. The flaking represents an inflammatory reaction to the natural yeast that lives on our scalp, though the reaction is more severe in some people than others. In fact, this yeast enjoys the oil that the scalp produces, meaning the scalp flaking can get worse when the scalp is more oily, not more dry. Occasionally, scalp flaking can lead to temporary hair loss, but this is rare and reversible.

The most common treatment for dandruff is dandruff shampoos, but guess what? These are often terrible options for those with curly hair. This is because they must be used daily for them to actually work. Tightly curly hair should be washed at most once a week. And just like using a lotion once a week won't help your dry skin, using a medicated shampoo once a week is often not enough. Also, most medicated shampoos are very drying. So, what do you do?

Well, fortunately, I have plenty of tips for controlling that stubborn dandruff in curly hair:

1. **Use a moisturizing shampoo designed for curly hair with zinc pyrithione** (see examples in Appendix B with product recommendations). Zinc pyrithione preparations tend to be more likely

to contain moisturizing ingredients than other dandruff shampoo products. However, it is still important to follow with a rich deep conditioner to minimize dryness.

2. **Wash your hair at least once a week.** Shampooing is an anti-inflammatory process and can help relieve symptoms. Going too long between shampoos will cause the flaking to get worse. This can be especially noticeable while wearing protective styles for extended periods of time without washing.

3. **Use a medicated steroid (or anti-fungal cream) a few times a week on itchy, scaly spots.** You can start with over-the-counter preparations, and if those don't work, talk to your dermatologist about a prescription-strength medication.

4. **If you are an essential oil fan, you can try diluted tea tree oil, which acts as a mild anti-inflammatory treatment.** Never apply undiluted essential oils directly to the scalp (see Chapter 43).

If all else fails, see a dermatologist! There are many prescription treatments for dandruff that are quite effective, and keeping this condition under control is key to protecting your healthy hair.

Forty-Eight

Recognize When Hair Loss May Be a Sign of Disease

It should go without saying that sometimes hair loss is your body's way of telling you that something is not right. If you have suddenly noticed that you are losing large clumps of hair every time you shower or brush your hair, this could be a sign that something is wrong. Many of the internal causes of hair loss are easily treatable and fortunately reversible, so you should not be afraid of talking to your doctor about your issues. Below are some common conditions found in women that can manifest as hair loss:

1. **Lupus:** This is an autoimmune condition in which the parts of your body that are designed to attack bacteria and viruses (your white blood cells) instead mistakenly begin to attack certain parts of your body. Patients with lupus will often complain of sudden sensitivity to sunlight, joint pains, and feeling unusually tired. Occasionally, they will also notice sudden hair loss that can leave bald patches. While lupus cannot be detected by routine bloodwork, your doctor can order more specialized bloodwork that can determine if you have lupus. In many women with tightly curled hair, severe disease can manifest as a loss in texture and curl pattern. For example, if you typically have coarse, tightly curled 4C hair, and over a matter of a couple of months, have noticed that your hair feels very fine with the curl pattern more like 3B or 3C, this could

be a sign of autoimmune disease (see Appendix C). In the setting of other symptoms—such as weight loss, fatigue, and some of the symptoms noted above—a full evaluation is warranted.

2. **Thyroid disease:** Like lupus, thyroid disease is often an autoimmune disease in which your body's cells attack the thyroid gland. Your thyroid gland is important for regulating your body's temperature, weight, and energy levels. Patients with thyroid disease may notice sudden hot flashes (not associated with menopause), rapid weight gain or loss, loss of energy, or feeling jittery. Any type of thyroid disease can lead to hair loss, typically manifesting as diffuse hair shedding. Women suffering from thyroid disease may notice a slow thinning all over the scalp or may notice large clumps of hair falling out while washing their hair. Thyroid disease is less likely to leave bald patches on the scalp. Since thyroid disease is so common among women, thyroid function is often checked during annual check-ups.

3. **Polycystic Ovarian Syndrome (PCOS):** This is a complicated disease that can be associated with infertility, severe acne, and hair loss. Women suffering from PCOS often have irregular periods, and the condition can cause weight gain. While women with PCOS will not necessarily notice hair shedding, they may notice their hair thinning over time, especially at the front and top of the scalp. PCOS is more difficult to diagnose because there is not a single blood test that confirms the diagnosis, but rather, having a specific set of symptoms in association with certain blood findings (including high testosterone levels) helps your doctor make the diagnosis. If you are concerned you may have PCOS, you can talk to your gynecologist about your symptoms and possible treatment options.

While these three conditions are some of the more common conditions that can lead to hair loss, many other conditions may cause it as well. It is important to make sure you are up to date on all of your health screenings. This is of critical importance not just for your hair health but your health in general.

Forty-Nine

Choose Hair Vitamins Carefully

Most of my patients are already on one or more supplements for hair growth by the time I see them for their first appointment. This is understandable as numerous companies have developed products claiming to boost hair growth, but do they measure up? Well, there are many things to consider when it comes time to select a vitamin for hair issues.

1. Indication: There are many dozen forms of alopecia, each of which requires a *unique* treatment approach. Think about it. Would you use your acne cream to treat your eczema just because they are both on the face? Just because two conditions are on the scalp, it does not mean the same treatment is effective for both. Most supplements/hair vitamins/herbals will claim to help alopecia without specifying if they are effective for any particular diagnosis.

2. Effectiveness: Supplements are not required to undergo any FDA testing to prove they work (they are considered "food" by the FDA), so only prescription medications require rigorous scientific data to prove effectiveness before they can be marketed for a condition. Almost no supplements (including beloved biotin) have been shown to be nearly as effective for ANY form of hair loss as medicated treatments such as minoxidil, which remains the gold standard treatment for many forms of non-scarring hair loss (see Chapter 46).

3. Safety: Similarly, absolutely no safety data is required for supplements to be sold, and companies are not required to report side effects. That means if clients suffer strokes, heart attacks, or worse, they are under no obligation to disclose these events unless enough clients *self-report* convincing claims to the FDA. Even then, the FDA may or may not act on this information. Prescription medications are required to pass rigorous safety thresholds *before* being sold or marketed. So, while side effects of supplements are unknown, rare and common side effects of prescription medications are reported and accessible to the provider or patient before use.

Okay, now that we have that out of the way, on to the fun stuff: Which vitamins actually work?

Well, researchers recently tackled this exact question and published their findings in the *International Journal of Dermatology* (see Appendix C). They found that the following vitamins have NO impact on any hair characteristics:

Biotin
Vitamin A
Vitamin D
Niacin
Selenium
Turmeric

Surprised? Many women swear by biotin even though there has never been any evidence that suggests it helps with hair health at all. They are more surprised to learn that the FDA has put out a warning against biotin, because taking it in supplemental doses can alter the values of many blood labs (see Appendix C). This has resulted in missed diagnoses that have led to deaths.

So, what vitamins do have some evidence of helping with the hair?

- **Iron** is helpful for those who are iron-deficient and suffering from sudden hair shedding. To enhance absorption, couple iron supplements with a source of vitamin C, like orange juice.
- **Zinc** supplementation may lead to improved regrowth in patients with a zinc deficiency, though zinc deficiencies are rare if you are following a normal diet.
- **Saw palmetto** can be effective for the treatment of age-related (i.e., female pattern) hair thinning. It works by blocking an enzyme called *5-alpha reductase*. This is the same enzyme that finasteride, a prescription medication approved for male pattern balding, targets. Because they work so similarly, the side effects are likely similar as well. Women with a history of breast cancer should consult with their physician before starting this hormonal supplement.
- **Marine complex powders** may lead to hair thickening, especially in those with age-related (female or male pattern) hair loss.
- **Pumpkin seed oil**, when taken by mouth, may improve female or male pattern hair loss as well.

So, there you have it. Keep in mind, all the studies in this article were small and limited, so more research has to be done to show definite benefits. However, if you insist on taking a supplement, drop the biotin in favor of one of these other supplements with better data supporting their use.

Finally, see a board-certified dermatologist to receive an accurate, timely diagnosis of your hair loss. If you decide to start a supplement, understand that the risks (and benefits) of supplement use are often unknown, even to your doctor, so proceed cautiously.

Fifty

See a Dermatologist for Hair Loss

As in the first book in this series, I have decided to end this book with this very important chapter. I hope that in reading this book you have learned a lot about what it takes to improve the health of your hair. For a few of you, however, this is less of a happy ending. If you have tried almost everything in this book, given it the requisite three months, and still notice issues with your hair, then I strongly recommend you see your dermatologist.

Dermatologists are specially trained at treating diseases of the skin, hair, and nails. There are at least a dozen different types of medical hair loss, and almost none can be reversed by what you have read in this book. While this book focuses on caring for the hair after it has left your scalp, a dermatologist can help you determine if you have a medical condition that is hindering hair growth. You should see a dermatologist if you are experiencing hair loss in the setting of scalp symptoms such as pain, burning, or itching in the scalp that doesn't seem to go away no matter what you try. The answer you are searching for may only be a doctor's visit away.

Appendix A

Sample Regimen

- Apply protein treatment to dry or damp hair. Cover with a shower cap or heating source for 30 minutes.
- Wash your hair once weekly with a sulfate-free shampoo.
- Deep condition with every shampoo. Follow deep conditioning with a moisturizing rinse-out conditioner. Alternatively, you could try a hot oil treatment.
- Add leave-in conditioner after washing, and at least three times a week.
- End your washing session with a light oil.

Other considerations

- Use sulfate-containing shampoo a maximum of once monthly.
- For severe damage, you could consider using stronger, salon-based protein treatments once monthly.
- Eliminate at least one damaging practice:
  o Air-dry hair whenever possible and limit blow-dry and flat-ironing to special occasions only.
  o Eliminate permanent color and switch to temporary rinses only until the damage is eliminated.
  o Eliminate the use of no-lye relaxers. Switch to texturizer or mild relaxers performed in salons only. Stretch relaxers to once every three months.

Appendix B

Product Recommendations

These product recommendations are based on personal experience and feedback from my patients. I do not have any financial relationships or endorse any of the listed brands. Remember, it may take a few tries before you find the product of your choice.

Shampoo: Sulfate-free ingredients to look for include cocomidopropyl betaine, decyl glucoside, and stearamidopropyl dimethylamine. This list also contains products with mild sulfates, like sodium C14-16 olefin sulfonate, which may interact more favorably with conditioners. *Avoid frequent use of shampoos with sulfates (sodium/ammonium lauryl sulfate, sodium/ammonium laureth sulfate, etc.)*

> TGIN Moisture Rich Sulfate Free Shampoo
> Crème of Nature Moisture & Shine Shampoo with Argan Oil
> Shea Moisture Raw Shea Butter Moisture Retention Shampoo
> NaturAll Avocado Shampoo with Kiwi
> Mielle Organics Pomegranate and Honey Shampoo
> Mielle Organics Babassu Conditioning Shampoo

Rinse-Out Conditioner:

> Aussie Moist Conditioner
> Hello Hydration Conditioner
> Tresemme Naturals Conditioner
> Crème of Nature Argan Oil Conditioner
> Trader Joe's Tea Tree Tingle Conditioner
> As I Am Coconut CoWash

Deep Conditioner

Pantene Gold Series Repairing Mask
Shea Moisture Manuka Honey & Mafura Oil Intensive Hydration Masque
Pantene Gold Series Moisture Renewal 3 Minute Miracle Deep Conditioner
Crème of Nature Argan Oil Intensive Conditioning Treatment
Aussie Moist 3 Minute Miracle
Organic Root Stimulator Olive Oil Replenishing Conditioner
Mielle Organics Rosemary Mint Strengthening Hair Masque
Mielle Organics Babassu Oil & Mint Deep Conditioner

Protein Treatments

Aphogee Keratin 2-minute Reconstructor
Shea Moisture Manuka Honey & Yogurt Power Protein Treatment
Olaplex Hair Perfector #3
Brigeo Don't Despair, Repair

Hair Oils (to be applied to wet hair)

Argan oil
Grapeseed oil
Jojoba oil
Olive oil
Coconut oil—best if used before or after shampooing

Leave-In Conditioners and Stylers

Luster's S Curl No Drip Activator
It's a 10 Miracle Leave-In
Cantu Shea Butter Leave-In Conditioning Cream

Melanin Hair Care Twist Elongating Style Cream
Camille Rose Naturals Almond Jai Twisting Butter
Kinky Curly Knot Today
Camille Rose Naturals Curl Maker
Alikay Naturals Shea Yogurt
As I Am So Much Moisture

Apple Cider Vinegar Rinses

Cantu Shea Butter Root Rinse
Girl + Hair Apple Cider Vinegar Clarifying Rinse

Anti-Dandruff Products

Head and Shoulders Royal Oils Line

Appendix C

Extra Reading

Benefits of Applying Coconut Oil to the Hair:
Gode V, N Bhalla, V Shirhatti, S Mhaskar, Y Kamath. "Quantitative mea-surement of the penetration of coconut oil into human hair using radiola-beled coconut oil." *Journal of Cosmetic Science.* Jan 1, 2012. 63(1):27–31.

Characteristics of Healthy Hair:
Sinclair RD. "Healthy hair: What is it?" *Journal of Investigative Dermatology.* Symposium Proceedings. Dec 1, 2007. (2): 12, 2–5. Elsevier.

Khumalo NP, PT Doe, RR Dawber, DJ Ferguson. "What is normal black African hair? A light and scanning electron-microscopic study." *Journal of the American Academy of Dermatology.* Nov 1, 2000. 43(5):814–20.

Essential Oils for Hair Growth:
Hay IC, M Jamieson, AD Ormerod AD. "Randomized trial of aromather-apy: Successful treatment for alopecia areata." *Archives of Dermatology.* Nov 1, 1998. 134(11):1349–52.

FDA Warning on Biotin
https://www.fda.gov/medical-devices/safety-communications/update-fda-warns-biotin-may-interfere-lab-tests-fda-safety-communication. Accessed March 1, 2022.

How Hair Products Work:
Bolduc C, J Shapiro. "Hair care products: Waving, straightening, condi-tioning, and coloring." *Clinics in Dermatology.* Jul 1, 2001. 19(4):431–6.

Side Effects Associated with Essential Oils

Henley DV, N Lipson, KS Korach, CA Bloch. "Prepubertal gynecomastia linked to lavender and tea tree oils." *New England Journal of Medicine.* Feb 2007. 1;356(5):479–85.

Mathew T, V Kamath, RS Kumar, M Srinivas, P Hareesh, R Jadav, S Swamy. "Eucalyptus oil inhalation–induced seizure: A novel, underrecognized, preventable cause of acute symptomatic seizure." *Epilepsia Open.* Sep 2017. 2(3):350–4.

de Groot AC, E Schmidt. "Tea tree oil: contact allergy and chemical composition." *Contact dermatitis.* Sep 2016. 75(3):129–43.

Linjawi SA. "Effect of camphor on uterus histology of pregnant rats." *Medical Science.* 2009.16(2).

https://www.hopkinsallchildrens.org/ACH-News/General-News/Are-Essential-Oils-Safe-for-Children. Accessed March 1, 2022.

Texture Changes due to Autoimmune Disease

Ajose FO. "Diseases that turn African hair silky." *International Journal of Dermatology.* Nov 2012. 51:12–6.

Traction Alopecia

Haskin A, C Aguh. "All hairstyles are not created equal: What the dermatologist needs to know about black hairstyling practices and the risk of traction alopecia (TA)." *Journal of the American Academy of Dermatology.* Apr 22, 2016.

Sung CT, ML Juhasz, FD Choi, NA Mesinkovska. The efficacy of topical minoxidil for non-scarring alopecia: a systematic review. *Journal of Drugs in Dermatology: JDD.* Feb 1, 2019. 18(2):155-60.

Vitamins and Supplements for Hair Loss

Gerkowicz A, K Chyl-Surdacka, D Krasowska, G Chodorowska. "The role of vitamin D in non-scarring alopecia." *International Journal of Molecular Sciences*. Dec 7, 2017. 18(12):2653.

Adelman MJ, LM Bedford, GA Potts. "Clinical efficacy of popular oral hair growth supplement ingredients." *International Journal of Dermatology*. Oct 2021.60(10):1199–210.

Looking for more in-depth scientific discussion of what you have read here? Then pick up my books:

Fundamentals of Ethnic Hair: The Dermatologist's Perspective, by Drs. Crystal Aguh and Ginette Okoye

90 Days to Beautiful Hair: 50 Dermatologist-Approved Tips to Un"lock" The Hair of Your Dreams by Dr. Crystal Aguh, U&C Publishing 2019°

Made in the USA
Columbia, SC
29 June 2022